TERESA SHI

G000075507

SWEET GRACE

HOW I LOST 250 POUNDS AND STOPPED TRYING TO EARN GOD'S FAVOR

"We have forgiveness for our failures based on His overflowing grace, which He poured over us with wisdom and understanding."

Ephesians 1:7b-8, Common English Bible

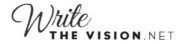

Write
THE VISION.NET

SWEET GRACE
HOW I LOST 250 POUNDS AND STOPPED TRYING TO EARN GOD'S FAVOR

Printed in the USA

ISBN: 978-0-9910012-0-0

Library of Congress Control Number: 2013951297

Published by Write the Vision | Columbia, Missouri   *Write* THE VISION.NET

Scripture taken from the Amplified® Bible is marked AMP. Copyright © 1954, 1958, 1962, 1964, 1965, 1987 by The Lockman Foundation. Used by permission.

Scripture taken from the Contemporary English Version is marked CEV. Copyright © 1995 American Bible Society. All rights reserved.

Scripture taken from the Good News Translation is marked GNT. Copyright © 1992 American Bible Society. All rights reserved.

Scripture taken from The Message ® is marked MSG. Copyright © 1993, 1994, 1995, 1996, 2000, 2001, 2002. Used by permission of NavPress Publishing Group. Colorado Springs, CO. All rights reserved.

Scripture taken from the New American Standard Bible® is marked NASB. Copyright © 1960, 1962, 1963, 1968, 1971, 1972, 1973, 1975, 1977, 1995 by The Lockman Foundation. Used by permission.

Scripture taken from the New English Bible: NET Bible® is marked NET. Copyright © 1996-2006 by Biblical Studies Press, L.L.C. http://netbible.com All rights reserved.

Scripture taken from the Holy Bible, NEW INTERNATIONAL READER'S VERSION® is marked NIRV. Copyright © 1996, 1998 Biblica. All rights reserved throughout the world. Used by permission of Biblica.

Scripture taken from the HOLY BIBLE, NEW INTERNATIONAL VERSION ® is marked NIV. Copyright © 1973, 1978, 1984 Biblica. Used by permission of Zondervan. All rights reserved.

Scripture taken from the New King James Version of the Bible is marked NKJV. Copyright © 1982 by Thomas Nelson, Inc. Used by permission. All rights reserved.

Scripture taken from the Holy Bible, New Living Translation is marked NLT. Copyright © 1996, 2004. Used by permission of Tyndale House Publishers, Inc., Wheaton, Illinois. All rights reserved.

To Contact the Author:

www.teresashieldsparker.com

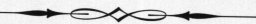

Teresa Shields Parker is a gifted writer and storyteller. *Sweet Grace* is the compelling story of one woman's journey into morbid obesity and out again. Teresa shares with warmth and honesty how she was able to confront her compulsive overeating and sugar addiction head on to find freedom in body, soul and spirit. As she learned to lose the excuses, stop hiding and face the truth, she was released to finally desire health and wholeness more than she craved sugar.

Throughout the book, Teresa encourages us to take action and make positive changes. Perhaps to this point, you have felt powerless to make the changes you know are essential to your freedom. As you read this book you'll discover how to tap into the power of the Holy Spirit who indwells us, always ready and available to help us clean up the mess of our lives. Get ready to find freedom and enter into the flow of God's unforced rhythms of grace!

—Dianne Wilson
Author, *Body & Soul*

SWEET GRACE

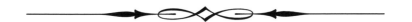

D E D I C A T I O N

To Roy, Andrew and Jenny who have loved me through
thick and thin, more of the former than the latter.
Where would I be without you?
You are each amazing examples of the
goodness, glory and grace of God in my life.

SWEET GRACE

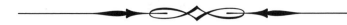

ACKNOWLEDGEMENTS

I t's hard to thank everyone who had a part in this book. I do want to give thanks to several who made the process go easier.

Thanks to my family and extended family for supporting me, loving me and putting up with me.

Thanks so much to my diligent first readers: Randy Shields, Renee Allen, Fran Hahn, Marilyn Logan, Lucie Winborne, Ruth West, Lorrie Ney, Linda Morris, Linda Ordway, Pamela Hodges and Becky Lusk. I can't thank you enough for your labor of love.

To my prayer group: I felt your prayers, every one of them, especially through the foggy and black as night times.

To the LOL girls: Your joyous laughter, heart-felt tears and deep love of God keep me sane in an insane world.

A special thanks to Wendy K. Walters, Aida Ingram and Karen Sinn, who are without a doubt coaches extraordinaire.

Above all, thanks to my heavenly Father. Despite my failures You never cease to pour out Your sweet grace on my mess of a life made beautiful because of You.

SWEET GRACE

AUTHOR'S NOTE

The stories, ideas and feelings expressed within this book are my perception of situations. Others may have a different interpretation or understanding of the same occurrences. In some chapters, names, characteristics or minor details have been changed or not included to protect the privacy of those I'd rather not name.

My immediate family members' names, as well as other friends and those who have helped me on the journey, are included. They have supported me in the decision to share my heart and my story, which at times has been hard. My husband said the story was difficult for him to read because it was like re-living things over again. However, he added he knew it was a story that will help others.

That's exactly the reason I wrote this book. I hope those who have gone through similar or related life experiences can connect the dots about how events in their lives may have impacted, especially in regard to losing weight, becoming healthy, maintaining relationships, working and overworking, living their dream and understanding God.

At the back of the book is a scripture section, which includes all the verses used in the study. This is for your quick reference or if you just have to read that scripture and can't find it in the book. Also included at the end of the book will be a link where you can go to my website and download the *Sweet Grace Study Guide* absolutely FREE. My gift to you.

The guide is designed to be used in your personal study. However, it would be easily adapted for a small group study. It is my prayer that you take time to download the study guide and use the questions to honestly ask yourself the questions and participate in the activities.

When I wrote the book, I wrote it with questions at the end of each chapter. It made more sense, though, to add to those and make a separate study guide.

However, the study guide is not just questions. It includes action steps to help you move towards your healthy life, creative activities, Bible Study questions, thought-provoking personal questions and ideas for developing a personal covenant.

We couldn't include very many photos in the book, so we included some in the study guide.

I wanted you to have access to the study guide. In order to download it at no charge go to www.teresashieldsparker.com/guide. Follow the prompts to download.

Print it, three-hole punch it and put it in a notebook. Use it to take notes as you read or if you want to contemplate what the chapter says, read the questions and do the activities together.

The study guide would also be a great tool to use for a small group study. Great conversation will be initiated as you share your journey and your discoveries from the book.

I wish I could be there to share your journey. I pray sweet grace as you walk this path.

—Teresa Shields Parker

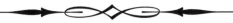

C O N T E N T S

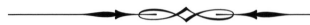

*"You saw me before I was born.
Every day of my life was
recorded in Your book.
Every moment was laid out
before a single day passed."*

Psalm 139:16 NLT

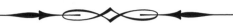

PROLOGUE

*"Oh unhappy and pitiable and wretched woman
that I am, who will release and deliver me from
[the shackles of] this body of death?"*

Romans 7:24, AMP

You walk into a friend's kitchen after having supper. Sitting on the counter is a plateful of warm brownies dotted with powdered sugar. Their smell wafts through the air filling the house. She encourages you to have as many as you want. You just finished supper about 20 minutes ago. Do you eat one or two, or more? Or since you just ate, do you decline the offer without a second thought?

For years my first response would be to eat as many as I could. And when she offered to send the rest home with me, I'd gladly oblige. It was unfathomable to me how my naturally thin husband would say, "No," in the same situation. If he was not hungry, no one could make him eat.

Today I make the choice easily not to eat brownies because I know they trigger a response in me that is difficult to stop. In the past, life revolved around food, the more the better. I told people I didn't know how I gained weight because I didn't eat that much. The truth was I had no idea how much I ate. I didn't keep track. I lived to eat.

Looking back at pictures of myself when I weighed 430 pounds, it's hard to understand who the person is staring back at me. I see the sadness in her eyes. The pain is visible. She doesn't know how to manage her appetite.

Rather than live with the difficulties of super morbid obesity, there was a time I felt it would be better if I was dead. And I wondered how I got to that point.

Sugar and bread were like drugs to me. I was addicted and couldn't stop eating. I loved God. I hated days of rage and days of weeping. I couldn't understand what was wrong with me. Why could I be successful in every other area except this one?

People who loved me wanted me to lose weight, but I rebelled against their caring advice. I felt they were treating me as a child. I was an adult. If I wanted to eat, I would eat. And so, eat I did.

Those who helped me the most didn't judge me. They simply asked what I wanted for my life. If I said that included being healthy, they would ask me how they could help. They offered help without judgment, which made me feel they really cared.

There are those who say, "Just eat less and exercise more." For those like me who constantly craved more and more food, it is too simplistic of an answer.

The majority of the population can eat and stop when they are full. But I can't, and perhaps you or your loved one can't either. It was not a matter of willpower. It was not a matter of being lazy. It was not a matter of being a heathen or ungodly.

Feeling "full" was a foreign concept to me. I was never full, even if I'd just eaten a meal. It is difficult to explain to those who do get full. But what if you never felt full? What if you were always and forever hungry?

What if there were mitigating circumstances that contributed to your weight gain? Things even you didn't understand? There is no easy solution. If so, obesity already would have been eradicated, but it is not, and you know it. You live with it every day.

Morbid obesity in any form is a living nightmare. I know. I was bound in chains of my own making. However, it need not feel like a solitary confinement sentence. You can break free.

I invite you to join me on my journey. If you are looking for a magic fix or immediate cure, you will not find it here. Believe me, I have tried all of them—including gastric bypass surgery. It worked in part until I began regaining the weight.

Any weight loss diet, supplement or surgery can be a tool to help lose weight. The real tool, though, was one I already had. I was the problem and I was the answer.

If you are morbidly obese, I am drawn to you because you desire so desperately to be set free. I see your misery. I see your despair. I see your pain. I see that you would rather not be encased in a body of death. I see your desire to be healthy. I see your craving to continue to eat. I see your desire to be anywhere, but in your own body.

Know this, God cares. He is not mad at you for running to food. He longs for you to come running into His arms of grace. He thinks you are beautiful. You are worthy. This is true whether you weigh 100 or 500 pounds. You are His trophy of grace when you submit totally to Him and His ways.

God's grace falls over us like the sweetness of sugar we've run to all our lives. We failed, yes, but God forgives failures because He's in the grace business. It's not just ordinary grace like we give a co-worker who takes our favorite pen. He gives us overflowing grace poured over us with wisdom and understanding when we turn away from our failures and towards Him.[1]

He understands your difficulties. He knows all about them. He has the wisdom to help you break free from the sugarcoated chains of morbid obesity.

There are answers. I found a way to gain control over what I felt powerless about. I invite you to bring an open mind and a heart full of courage for yourself and those you love as you join me in traveling through God's sweet grace that brings power for breaking the sugarcoated chains that have bound and shackled you in life-long misery.

ENDNOTES

1. Ephesians 1:7b-8, CEB

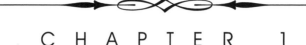
SWEET GRACE

"For it is by grace you have been saved, through faith—and this is not from yourselves, it is the gift of God—not by works, so that no one can boast."

Ephesians 2:8-9 NIV

Friday nights were always the same: grocery store, then laundromat. One particular Friday night, though, looms in my mind as life changing. My brother and I were behaving as well as could be expected. We didn't run screaming through the aisles. At the checkout stand we eagerly waited for the dimes Dad gave us for being good. We would use them to buy penny candy.

"I'm sorry," Dad said. "I don't have enough dimes to share with you. I barely have enough to get the laundry done. Things are tight this week." He patted us both on the shoulder and turned to help Mom.

My brother didn't seem too concerned. He was driving his little metal car around an imaginary racetrack.

I, however, was angry. I wanted my candy. I deserved my candy. I had been good. I had done what I was told and now I deserved to have candy. I looked at the penny candies. There were Tootsie Rolls®, caramels and all my seven-year-old favorites.

It was too simple, really. It was right there. The right hand quickly took a handful of penny candies and stuck them in the large pocket of my vinyl jacket. It was mindless, as if I wasn't even involved in the activity. All of sudden, the candy just appeared in my coat pocket. I was happy. I had what I "deserved".

NOT SHARING

All the way to the laundromat, the candy called to me. I couldn't stand it. I had to eat one. I stuck my hand in the pocket and one-handedly unwrapped a Tootsie Roll®. I thought to myself, "How clever of me to be able to accomplish such a feat." I made sure the candy stayed hidden in my hand as I quickly popped it in my mouth.

It must have been the chocolate aroma that alerted my little brother. He looked at me. I knew he knew.

"I want some," he said.

My parents were talking in the front seat of the loud Plymouth. They couldn't hear us.

"No, these are mine." I popped another in my mouth.

"I want one."

"No." I unwrapped a caramel and chewed it slowly.

I was brazen. I should have known better. I should have given up one of the stolen morsels.

Randy watched as I put the last piece of buttery sweetness in my mouth. Now he wouldn't get any of my candy. There was none left. When I showed him it was all gone that was the last straw.

"Mommy, Sissy didn't give me any of her candy."

"Teresa, where did you get candy?" Mom looked over her glasses. "Did you give her money, Ernie?"

Dad shook his head no.

"Teresa Kay, did you steal that candy?" Mom pressed for an answer.

I couldn't bring myself to speak. I hadn't thought of what I had done as stealing. The candy was there. I wanted it. I deserved it. I took it. It wasn't stealing like a bank robber steals. It was just penny candy.

Dad told me to wait in the car. He helped Mom inside with the laundry and then came out. Silently we drove back to the store.

CONFESSION

We walked into the familiar market and up to the customer service booth.

"We need to see the manager," Dad said. His voice was quiet.

We walked up the stairs to Charlie's office. It had a big picture window where he could see everything. I had never realized that's where his office was. Now I was worried. Did he see me take the candy?

I knew who Charlie was. Dad would stop and make small talk with him from time-to-time. However, I could tell this was not to be a casual conversation.

"My daughter has something to tell you," Daddy said.

My father's eyes bore a hole in me and waited for a confession. I hadn't realized I had something to tell him until that very moment.

"I stole some candy," I said hanging my head.

"How much candy?" Charlie asked.

I glanced up to see him concentrating on me. I dropped my head again.

"Four pieces."

"Stealing anything, even candy, is a crime," he said with a grave tone in his voice. "You could be arrested. Do you know what happens when people are arrested?"

I nodded my head yes.

"Tell me," he said.

"They go to jail?" I said.

"Yes, they can."

"Oh," I was genuinely scared at this point. I'd stolen candy before from a stash in the cabinet. Since my parents had already paid for any candy I'd ever taken from them, I didn't figure it was really stealing. Today was my first criminal act and I had been caught.

"Do you still have the candy?" he asked.

I shook my head no. Truth was my only resource. Mercy was my only hope.

"Do you have money to pay for what you took?"

Again, I shook my head no.

"Do you have anyone who can bail you out of this? Anyone you can borrow the money from?"

My heart pounded. My father's eyes were soft. "Daddy, can I borrow the money? I don't want to go to jail."

My father handed me a dime. I turned it over in my hand. I worried that one load of laundry might not get dry because of my indiscretion. Even so, I gave Charlie the coin. He took it, but his eyes never left mine.

"I want you to promise me you will never steal again. I will not look the other way next time. Your father is a good man. Do what he tells you."

"Yes, Sir." I knew going to the grocery store would never be the same again.

I AM A SINNER

Walking to the car, Daddy took my hand. I looked up at his creased face and saw a tear trickle down his cheek.

For the first time, it hit me. I am the sinner the pastor preaches about. My earthly father knows it and my heavenly Father knows it. I deserve punishment.

That night I didn't know what to call it, but I felt driven, compelled to pray a child-like sinner's prayer. "Jesus, I'm a sinner. Forgive me. Come into my heart. Save me from hell."

That's pretty much all I was after. I wanted fire insurance. I got grace.

I didn't understand that I had a weakness, an all-consuming pull towards sweets, which would at some point seek to replace God in my life. Yet, in the moment of coming to Him, He forgave what would become my obsession. He knew one day I would recognize, repent and run to Him for my needs instead of going to what my body craved.

After that day whenever I had temptation to steal I easily ignored it. That, however, was not the case with eating sugar. I became addicted, plain and simple. I belonged to God, but this weakness nearly took me under. It would have, had it not been for His sweet grace gently supporting me and calling me back time and time again.

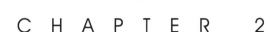

TOO BIG FOR MY HEART

"Today I have given you the choice between life and death, between blessings and curses. I call on heaven and earth to witness the choice you make. Oh, that you would choose life, that you and your descendants might live! Choose to love the Lord your God and to obey Him and commit yourself to Him, for He is your life. Then you will live long in the land the Lord swore to give your ancestors Abraham, Isaac, and Jacob."

Deuteronomy 30:19-20, NLT

How did I get to this point in my life? I was in the hospital waiting for the results of an angiogram to see what type of heart surgery I needed. My weight was somewhere between gigantic and humongous.

The more pressing problem was rolling over on my side in what felt like the world's smallest hospital bed. I had an I.V. stuck in my left arm. With my right hand I reached across and grabbed the left bed rail and tried to pull myself on to my side.

Gradually, grudgingly the mountain of flesh, which had become my body, complied. In slow motion my belly waved forward. With awkward movement, I hefted my right leg onto my left. My hips didn't seem to want to comply.

"Can I help you?" The student nurse bounced into the room.

"Just trying to get on my side." She stared as if she had never seen a 430-pound woman try to turn over in a twin bed. I felt like a science experiment gone bad as the rest of my body refused to budge.

"Maybe if I pushed from the other side?" She became a blur as she sped around the bed. I glowered although she couldn't see the expression on my face. She positioned her hands on the mountain of my rump.

"On the count of three, you pull on the rail and I'll push. One. Two. Three."

She straightened the covers and pulled them over me. Adjusting the pillows she chatted away about what a nice day it was outside and how good it must feel for me to change positions. She took my temperature, blood pressure and checked the I.V. bag.

Coming back to the bedside, she patted my arm in a matronly sort of way. "What else can I get you?" She sounded just like the window clerk at the fast food drive-through I frequented.

"How about two double cheeseburgers, large fries and an extra-large Diet Coke®?" I shouldn't have said it, I know, but I just couldn't resist.

For one brief second I saw her eyebrows furrow into a frown. "Oh, you were joking, right? I can get you a diet cola and some peanut butter crackers. How would that be?"

"Just the diet. Don't want to spoil my girlish figure." She didn't laugh. She was gone quicker than I could say, "Wait, I changed my mind." After all, it was a whole hour before breakfast. I sighed. I was hungry, but then I was always hungry.

THE ISSUE

She returned with the soda just as the intern with intense blue eyes walked in. His dark hair curled around the collar of his white lab coat. "Your urine output is awesome." Not a very good line for such a handsome young man.

He continued, "The Lasix is really working well. By the time you are out of here you will be thin and trim." He laughed. In my mind he fell at least three steps down from movie star status.

"Just keep up the good work." How could I do anything else? Lasix, the medication being pumped into me intravenously, was draining the fluid from around my heart. The fluid was expelled straight into the catheter. I had nothing to do with the process.

"Do you know what the angiogram showed?" I asked.

"The cardiac surgeon will be in sometime this morning to give you all the results. It looked fine."

"How could it look fine? I need a heart valve replacement. That's not fine."

"I'll let the surgeon tell you all about it." He, too, patted my arm. I wanted to pull it away. I was not a dog or a small child.

13

"I want to know. I'm the patient here. I should know." I became acutely aware my voice raised several notches. I needed an answer and I could be no-nonsense in order to get it.

He leaned forward as if he were going to reveal a secret and then stopped when he heard the heart surgeon talking to a nurse outside the door. His eyes darted that direction. "I need to join the entourage in the hall for morning rounds."

SURGERY

They had started me on Lasix in anticipation of surgery. I would need open-heart surgery to replace the valve and possibly remove blockages. The angiogram would show exactly what they were dealing with. At the most it would be a valve replacement and bypass and at the least, a valve replacement.

At my size, any surgery was risky, but especially open heart surgery. I couldn't help but remember my father's surgery several years earlier. They did four bypasses. He had been a little overweight at the time of surgery and had high blood pressure. He did like to eat, especially sweets.

After his surgery, only one family member at a time was allowed in the recovery room. His skin reminded me of chalk, pasty white. He was hooked up to what seemed like a myriad of wires. It was freezing in the room. He looked dead. He had a cannula for oxygen, so I knew he was breathing. My brain argued that he might just be kept alive to harvest his organs. I tried to stop the wayward thoughts. I didn't want to think about life without him.

I wondered if he would pull through the recovery process. After all, they cut open his chest, spread apart his ribs, deflated and then re-inflated his lungs and played with his heart. That didn't seem like something a person could survive and come out better after it was over.

Leaving the room, I was visibly shaken. My brother met me in the hall. "He looks dead, doesn't he?" I nodded my head fighting back tears. I couldn't speak. He stopped and turned to face me.

"I think I'm going to go get a stress test done," he said. "This has made me think I need to take better care of myself."

"Maybe I will too," I said still remembering the picture of my dad in the cold room.

"Good." He waited until I looked up at him. "I don't want to have to visit you here." He motioned to the recovery room. "Know what I mean?" I nodded my head yes, but couldn't stop the tears from escaping. He gave me a hug.

I knew it had been hard for him to say the words. I also knew he meant them from the depths of his heart. I vowed to do better. I did do better. I went on one of the many diets I had been on through the years. This time it was a high protein diet. I ate meat and very few carbohydrates. I severely limited my food intake with a goal of losing 100 pounds. I knew I could do it because I had done it before.

When I accomplished that feat, it felt good. I was proud. So I rewarded myself by going off the diet and resuming my old habits, which consisted of eating whatever I wanted, whenever I wanted.

It didn't take long to gain 100 pounds back. My body always seemed maniacal to me in that it would not only gain the weight back, but also add about 30 pounds. It happened every time I went off a diet and started eating regular food. I couldn't seem to stop myself. I hated the way I looked. But plain and simple, I had a love affair with food, the sweeter, richer, fatter, more bread-heavy, the better.

REGULAR PHYSICIAN ASSESSMENT

After gaining the weight back for what seemed like the millionth time, I decided to just accept myself fat and all. I went to my regular physician. She assured me I didn't have diabetes or high blood pressure, both of which ran on both sides of my family.

"As far as symptoms, you don't have any right now." The woman doctor looked at me waiting to make eye contact, but I looked at my shoes.

Short and a little overweight, she continued. "While it is true most people of your weight would have multiple health problems, it is good news you don't have them so far. I am concerned, though, that you could develop these down the road. I would suggest a low-fat diet." She handed me a standard food pyramid print out with low-fat choices.

She smiled at me. "I have issues with weight, so I know a little of what you are going through. Even if you just lost a few pounds it would benefit your overall health."

"I can lose weight." I looked her in the eyes mainly because there didn't seem to be anything else interesting in the small room. "I have lost tons of weight over the years, but I always gain it back plus more. I hate the yo-yo dieting."

She nodded. "Diets never work. It has to be a lifestyle change. Losing weight and gaining it back is not optimal for your body. There are no good and bad foods. It helps to manage your portions and make healthier choices."

I knew what she was telling me. If I wasn't planning on changing the way I ate for the rest of my life, it would be more detrimental for me to keep losing and re-gaining. My body would give out from the stress of constant change.

DIETS DON'T WORK

I walked out and threw the handout in the trashcan. I had a closet full of weight loss supplements. I'd been on every diet including ones that cost lots of money like Diet Center® and Nutri-Systems®. I'd been on ones that cost very little or no money like low fat, low calorie, high protein, low carbohydrate, no carbohydrate, grapefruit and who knows what else.

All were the same. All of them worked as long as I stayed with the plan. I'd stay on them for a while and lose weight. Then I'd breathe a sigh of relief and go back to the way I always ate. Before long, I'd gain it back plus more.

If I didn't have specific health issues, then why do that to myself? Sure, I couldn't walk across the super center, but I could sit, rest, get up and go again. I could manage.

PRAYING

Today, though, the health issues monster had caught me. In a matter of a few days it would devour me with a knife and scalpel. I wanted to know what would happen, when it would happen and how it would happen. I wanted to know every detail so I could worry, fret, pray, worry and fret some more.

Many times I had actually prayed, "Lord, make me thin. Lord, take away my cravings for donuts, cinnamon rolls, candy, oatmeal cookies, chocolate cake with coconut and pecan icing, chicken fried steak with gravy and homemade bread. Thank you, in Jesus' name. Amen."

That type of praying sent me to the kitchen to whip up a batch of whatever sounded the best. I always came to the same conclusion. "I am doomed to be fat. I will always be fat. It is my cross to bear. It is my lot in life. I might as well accept it." So I did.

> I am doomed to be fat. I will always be fat. I might as well accept it.

I knew I should pray, "Lord, give me strength to resist things I shouldn't eat. Help me understand the things which are best for me." That kind of prayer, though, would require me to do some hard work. It might also require I participate in that horrible eight-letter word—exercise. I shuddered just thinking about it.

I might look stupid with a body more than twice the size necessary, but I knew what it took to lose weight. I knew I would need to eat healthy for the rest of my life. I knew I would need to exercise regularly. That didn't sound like fun—it sounded like torture!

Eating provided recreation and distraction for me. It had become my source of fun. To do without eating my favorite comfort foods would mean giving up the main enjoyment in my life. I didn't want to do that, not forever. I could do it short-term, but short-term diets turned into long-term extreme weight gain for me. So my decision was not to do it at all.

If I had examined my thinking in detail, I would have seen it was ridiculously flawed. Many times my friends, family members and I had consoled each other with words like, "If we were only alcoholics, then we could just stay away from alcohol and be cured. Alas, we love to eat and a person can't stay away from food. We have to eat."

I'd even said I would rather be dead than not be able to eat what I wanted. If I continued to eat for three people, I might get my wish.

FIVE YEARS TO LIVE

No fewer than 10 men and women, dressed in white lab coats, descended on my bed like a plague. They reminded me of a group of human-sized praying mantises waiting to grab me and tear me to shreds. (Of course, a praying mantis cannot tear apart a human, but I detest their beady eyes and front feet that look like they could.)

Although the intern hadn't given me the information I wanted, I focused on him because he was easy to look at. The surgeon nodded to him to give the run-down on me.

He rattled off my statistics. "45 year-old female, five foot, five inches, 430 pounds, presents with super morbid obesity, high blood pressure, diabetes, mitral valve prolapse and trouble breathing."

Wait. Time out. Rewind. That's not me. You must have gotten the records mixed up. I wanted to shout, jump out of bed, grab the "movie star" by his white lapels and shake some big screen sense into him.

I don't have diabetes or high blood pressure. And what's this term "super morbid" they tacked on? I mean, sure I was obese. I knew that. The word morbid, though, conjured up scenes of a ghastly Halloween portrayal of a graveyard complete with casket and flying bats. I was still alive. With the word "super" I heard, "Do you want to super-size that?" I looked down at my body and silently, I said, "Sure, why not?"

The intern continued, "Patient had an angiogram yesterday morning. Results show no mitral value prolapse, no obstructions. However, there is significant fluid build-up in the ventricular cavity."

I looked around the room trying to read the faces. I definitely needed a translation. "What does all that mean?"

The cardiac surgeon had olive skin and black hair. He was articulate with a slight accent. He was said to be a world-renowned cardiologist, but he was devoid of a bedside manner and didn't sugarcoat anything.

"You have congestive heart failure," he said. "Your body is too big for your heart. Your heart was never designed to support a body of your current weight. You need to lose at least 100 pounds. You need to do it now or you will be dead in five years. You need gastric bypass surgery. We do it here. My nurse will set you up with an appointment."

He turned and walked out of the room. The intern looked at me with sad eyes. The others averted theirs from the spectacle in front of them as they hurried to catch up with the renowned heart surgeon who was already asking for particulars on the next patient.

"I'll be by later to explain things to you," the intern said as he left the room.

What is there to explain, I wondered? I am fat. I am going to die. It's pretty self-explanatory. I'm a smart girl. I get what this means.

STOP EATING OR DIE

The hospital bustled with morning activity. Patient bells rang out at the nurse's station. Monitors beeped for attention. The noise seemed to fade in oblivion. I placed my hand over my chest just to make sure. Yes, I was alone, just me and my heart.

Dad's heart was repaired with a quadruple bypass. Mine couldn't be repaired in any way except to stop food from going into my mouth. It was much simpler than open-heart surgery, but it didn't seem that way at the time.

I began to run through my options. I had a friend in college who had her stomach stapled. Of course that was when the surgery was new. Recently, I'd read about the new version called Roux-En-Y Gastric Bypass surgery. There were several things I didn't like about it. For starters, the small metal ring placed around the esophagus concerned me. What if food got stuck there? Would it require another surgery?

A portion of the stomach was cut off and a small pouch constructed. The smaller stomach is connected directly to the middle portion of the small intestine, called the jejunum, passing the rest of the stomach and the upper part of the small intestine called the duodenum. Because of bypassing a portion of the small intestine, patients have to take daily vitamins and minerals for the rest of their lives. They will not absorb all the nutrients they need from food. Eating large quantities, at least at first, is no longer possible.

I had heard the surgery wasn't safe and had a high mortality rate. If I were going to die, I might as well die happy with food in my rather large belly.

Another option occurred to me, though. I could go on the high protein diet again. I lost 100 pounds on it two times actually. Of course, I had gained it back, but I could lose it again. I'd have to be more careful this time. I'd have to stick with the plan for a longer time.

LIFE WOULD END

It's interesting how aware I became of my heart when there was a possibility it could stop at any time. I could be picking up my teenager at high school, watching my daughter sing with her fifth grade honors choir and it would be too much. My heart would stop. Life would end. I would not be able to see them grow up, graduate high school and college, get married and do all the awesome things I knew they would do. I'd miss their lives. I'd miss their children's lives.

My husband would do the best job he could with them. He'd do great with Andrew. He'd try his best with Jenny. Children, though, especially daughters, need their mother. Andrew was 15. Jenny was only eight. They had their whole lives ahead of them. They were too young to lose me.

Would they remember me? Andrew barely remembered my mother and she had died only six years before. What kind of legacy would I leave them? Should I write a book? Leave them a videotape? What about my husband? How could I miss growing older with him?

Then there was our mentally challenged foster son. He had been living with us for about seven months. The rejection of moving so soon would be hard for him. Worse than all of these things, though, I'd miss my life. I still had things to do. I had women to coach. I had small groups to lead. I had foster children to raise. I had articles, publications and books to write. I wasn't done yet. I had visions of the future, didn't I?

I always said I wanted to lose weight. I mean what morbidly obese person really wants to weigh over 400 pounds?

PLEADING WITH GOD

I screamed inside. "Why does this have to happen to me?"

I cried. "I don't deserve this."

I pleaded with God to be able to wake up and realize this was all a bad dream and I weighed a normal weight or at least had no weight issues.

I don't ever remember being in shock before. That day I was in shock. My mouth hung open. My eyes had an expressionless stare. I was going to die.

I had lived my life expecting something magical to happen to me. One day I would wake up and no longer want to eat as much. Or maybe I'd go through a healing line and all of a sudden before everyone's eyes 250 pounds or more would disappear from my body like the incredible shrinking woman. I would go on a speaking tour, telling everyone how great God is that He did this miracle in my life. No matter how hard I prayed, though, the miracle did not happen.

Now here I was with an extreme problem. If I had faith, I could say to the mountain (of flesh) move and it would move.[1] Obviously, I didn't have that kind of faith.

I had gotten to this point on my own volition, sweet morsel by sweet morsel, each one a conscious adult choice.

RUDE CARDIAC SURGEON

Somewhere during that day, I made a decision to live. I guess I owe my life to a rude cardiac surgeon who made me realize I really do want all life has to offer. He helped me understand there are no magic cures, only intentional actions. I seriously doubt he ever read the Bible. He just didn't appear to be that kind of guy. However, I believe he would agree with what Moses told the children of Israel.

"Today I have given you the choice between life and death, between blessings and curses. I call on heaven and earth to witness the choice you make. Oh, that you would choose life, that you and your descendants might live! Choose to love the Lord your God and to obey Him and commit yourself to Him, for He is your life. Then you will live long in the land the Lord swore to give your ancestors Abraham, Isaac, and Jacob"[2]

The mandate was clear. My choice was a no-brainer. I chose life. Grabbing it with both hands, however, was still years away. Finally I knew the truth. My compulsive overeating had limited me and pronounced a death sentence over my life. The original question still remained. How did I get to this point and what was I going to do about it?

ENDNOTES

1. Matthew 17:20, NIV
2. Deuteronomy 30:19-20, NLT

SWEET GRACE

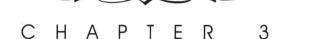

COMFORT FOOD

"Now we see things imperfectly, like puzzling reflections in a mirror, but then we will see everything with perfect clarity. All that I know now is partial and incomplete, but then I will know everything completely, just as God now knows me completely."

1 Corinthians 13:12, NLT

To an 18-month-old the bag of white balls under the cabinet resembled candy, not really marshmallows, but close. Maybe gum balls? I had to find out. I had eaten two of them before Mom caught me and panicked. She grabbed me and ran to the neighbor's house breathlessly explaining I had eaten mothballs.

"Do you think they are poisonous?" she asked.

Her friend didn't know, but a quick phone call to the local hospital and they were on the way to the emergency room with me. Dad took off work and met them there. They were mortified. I was their only child.

Just a few months earlier Mom had lost a little girl. The baby was stillborn. The hospital staff did not tell my parents right away about the baby's death, making the news even harder to take. She and Dad weren't allowed to see or hold the baby.

My father had to drive his stillborn daughter from Texas to Missouri in a little box. She was buried in Fayette. Papaw, my mother's father, bought seven burial plots in the cemetery so the baby would not be alone. Mom, Dad, Grandma and Papaw are buried with her today. So perhaps the plan worked.

START OF EMOTIONAL SLIDE

Shortly after the baby was buried, my father's father passed away so my dad stayed in Missouri longer than he thought he would. My mother's mother had come to help ease the burden for Mom. She stayed as long as necessary.

No matter how long Grandma stayed, though, she couldn't help Mom get over the baby's death. It hit Mom hard. It was the beginning of times when she escaped into a land of nothingness. It would get worse as she got older and she had more children. During this time, though, she was coping as best she could.

We lived in a silver Airstream travel trailer. It had a lean-to built on one side as a living room. My father was in Bible college in Texas, so the mobile home was in a student housing area. The trailer was tiny. One couldn't turn around without bumping into a piece of furniture or another person. That's why I believe Mom, even at this point in time, was in her thought world and didn't notice what I was doing or what I was eating.

My stomach was pumped and everything turned out fine. Mom told the story many times because I gave her such a scare. The story sticks in my mind because it involves me eating something I must have thought was candy. It was a tendency I had even as a toddler.

As most kids, I loved anything with sugar, especially candy. The concentrated sugar content made me feel better, like everything was right with the world when most of the time everything was not right with my world, at least from my perspective as the oldest child.

SUPPERTIME

When I was growing up, supper at our house was very regimented, partly due to a limited budget. If Mom cooked, she would prepare just enough for one portion for each. Dessert would usually be a can of fruit cocktail divided between us. When my little sister came along, we'd divide two cans among five.

Mom was very big on having a meat, a fruit, a vegetable and a starch, such as potatoes or noodles, with our meals. In other words, she tried hard to serve balanced meals. Most of the time the meat would be fish sticks, hamburger or hot dogs. Every once in awhile we would have pork chops or roast, but only if Papaw had given us the meat.

My father's contribution to the meal was two-fold. He insisted we always say grace. He told us stories of how at times he and his four brothers and sister did not have anything to eat in the house except a jar of canned cherries. They would have that for supper. His father was an alcoholic farmhand. My dad knew what going without food was like and wanted to be sure we were thankful for what we had.

His other contribution was his signature laugh and the twinkle in his eyes. He asked us about our day. We took turns going around the table telling what happened at school or with our friends. It was the main time I felt connection with my family. The other special time for me was when I would go with my Dad to church on a Wednesday night, just the two of us.

CARAMEL THIEF

Sneaking snacks was forbidden. That constituted a belt spanking. Still I risked the beating to sneak caramels from the bag Mom kept on the top shelf in the kitchen. The kitchen cabinets were tall, at least to a small child.

In order to reach the candy, I had to pull a chair over to the counter, stand on the chrome-legged chair, climb up on the Formica countertop, stand up, open the door past me balancing so I didn't fall and reach way back in the corner. It was not an easy feat, but so worth it if I could get away with it. Most of the time, Mom was in her bedroom, which was about as far from the kitchen as it got in our small house.

I had been successful swiping candy on many occasions. Then I got braver and started taking more pieces at once. One day I had taken all the candy left in the bag (which was several pieces). Mom was asleep. I didn't think anything about sitting on the gray tile kitchen floor and unwrapping each piece. I closed my eyes and savored the taste as it melted in my mouth.

I was taken to another place with each bite of sugary, buttery, creamy ecstasy where everything was perfect and I had all the candy I wanted. I was shocked when I opened my eyes and she was staring at me, hands on her hips, legs apart in a fighter's stance. Needless to say, I got a sound spanking. She was very upset that I had disobeyed, but the real anger was because I had eaten her last piece of candy.

From then on she hid the caramels in her room. Every once in awhile, she would give me a few pieces as a reward when I cleaned the entire house or did all the laundry. I would do almost anything for a caramel.

CANDY ON THE BRAIN

I lived for Halloween mainly because we got gobs of candy, a pillowcase full. I really didn't like dressing up or wearing the hot plastic mask that fogged my glasses. I didn't like going up to doors and hearing spooky music. I didn't like people asking me what trick I'd do if they didn't give me a treat. I endured it all for one reason and one reason only—candy. There were never any limits placed on how much candy we could eat. Mine was always gone by the next day. And I wished I had more.

Christmas, Valentine's Day and Easter were other special occasions when we got and could eat all the candy we wanted. Whatever I got was not enough. I craved more. I had candy on the brain most of the time. Any money I got went to buy my favorites, which included anything with caramel, chocolate, peanut butter, fruit flavors and nuts. Pretty much any candy would do.

MOM'S SICKNESS

Renee, my sister, was born when I was eight. She was a beautiful, blonde-haired delight to us all. Mom had become increasingly more distant and moody. Having three children in a small, five-room house could not be a walk in the park, especially for someone who had emotional issues already.

I remember Mom being physically present, but not really being there. She would stare off into another world for hours, sitting almost catatonic. At other times she would be angry and yelling. Then some days she would be perfectly normal.

If you asked her about what happened the day before, she would act as if she didn't know what you were talking about. Sometimes I wondered if I had dreamed what happened. If so it would have been in the nightmare category.

I never knew what kind of mother I would come home to when school was over. By this time, Randy was in school, as well. She seemed to be able to take care of my sister during the day until Renee was old enough to go to school.

> I never knew what kind of mother I would come home to when school was over.

There were also times when Mom went into the psychiatric ward at the local hospital, into a mental health facility in our town or into the state mental hospital. Many of these times seemed to be in the summers. I would watch my siblings during the day and take care of everything a mother was supposed to do.

There were things I didn't know how to do, couldn't know how to do. I tried to keep up with my brother and sister. I did laundry. I cleaned. I cooked. I washed dishes. I helped Dad buy the groceries because he had no idea what to buy. He worked all day, but he helped as much as he could after work. He had a huge weight on his shoulders just trying to keep everything and everyone together.

When I asked Dad what was wrong with Mom, he would say, "She is sick." That became what I told others if they asked. Of course I knew she was not sick with the flu or a cold. There was something else going on with her. I just wasn't sure what.

PAPAW'S PRAYER

When I was 12 years old, Mom went into the state mental hospital. It was during the summer. The weekend after she went in the hospital, Dad took us to Grandma's house and left us for the weekend. My grandparents were sitting at the kitchen table when I walked in the house. I pulled up a red vinyl chair and sat down. Running my finger along the chrome molding on the white metal table, I told them what it had been like the week before Mom went into the hospital.

"She cried all day long. And then she started talking about very strange things. It scared me because I didn't know what she meant. I really couldn't figure out what she was saying, but I knew I hadn't done whatever it was. She was really mad. Then she sat and stared. What's the matter with her?"

I looked at Papaw. He took my hand and shook his head. "I don't know. I just don't know." He swiped at the water in the corners of his eyes. I started to cry. I couldn't help it. I'd never seen Papaw cry before. Grandma took my other hand. She didn't say a word, but the tears were rolling down her cheeks, as well.

Then Papaw prayed for Mom, me and the rest of the family. I had heard Papaw pray for the meal and I had heard him pray with Grandma before they went to sleep at night. But I'd never heard him pray in the middle of the day, especially for me. He prayed for God to keep me safe and comfort me. He prayed that God would touch my mother and heal her.

Later Grandma said, "I don't know why she's like this. I worry we did something wrong raising her. But she had a great life." Then taking my chin in her hands she said, "If you ever need me, you call me."

I nodded my head yes, but I wouldn't call. I would get spanked for calling her long-distance. I would get spanked if Mom thought I had told Grandma anything about how she acted. She didn't want Grandma to know she had a problem. She had even said she didn't want Grandma and Papaw to come visit her in the hospital.

"Can't I just come live with you forever?" I asked.

"I have to leave that up to your daddy. You're the oldest. The best help you can be to your daddy is to be there and help with things. I can't be there, but you can. I'm counting on you."

GRANDMA'S HOUSE

While I was at Grandma's the contrast was so real I could touch it. Grandma and I worked, but we worked together. When I was at home, I had to do everything by myself.

Grandma worked all day long. She got up early to get Papaw's breakfast and fixed him a large lunch and supper. Papaw farmed, doing the planting and harvesting. He also took care of the livestock, which included cows, pigs, sheep and horses.

Grandma's main morning chore after breakfast involved gathering the eggs. I didn't like this chore because the setting hens had to be moved off the nests. Most of the time, they protested making all kinds of noises, as well as trying to peck me.

Papaw would bring the milk in about mid-morning. Grandma would strain it, separating the cream from the milk. Then she put both in the refrigerator. Once a week she'd churn butter from the cream. Her churn was electric, but still difficult to handle. She put the cream in with a little salt, turning it on and holding the churn so it didn't dance all over the counter top.

Although I tried to help with this process a time or two, I couldn't hold the churn still and had to yell for Grandma to help before it fell off the counter. After churning, Grandma would pat the butter into a mold. The liquid left was buttermilk. Papaw loved butter-churning day because he'd eat cornbread and buttermilk for supper. I didn't understand how he could stand it, but he loved it.

Grandma planted a huge garden. There was always something to pick, pull, dig, break or hull. Green beans, lima beans, peas, okra, corn, tomatoes, carrots, onions, potatoes and turnips were included in the large assortment in her garden. Most summer evenings, the task was shelling peas or breaking green beans while sitting in the dark green metal lawn chairs under the big oak tree in the front yard.

Certain days were set aside for killing and dressing chickens. I watched as the process was done from start to finish, but never really got the hang of any part of it except the cooking and eating. Grandma made the world's best fried chicken, gravy, mashed potatoes and hot rolls.

OATMEAL COOKIES

Making oatmeal cookies with my grandmother was the closest I ever came to heaven here on earth. From the time I was a toddler, I can remember standing in a chair pulled up to the kitchen counter and helping her stir the ingredients for cookies. It was her special recipe, which I've since taught to my daughter. I thought for many years it was our secret, Grandma's and mine. In actuality, it's an easy recipe that's in most every cookbook.

By the time I was eight, I had memorized the recipe and could make the cookies at home. Making them with Grandma, though, was always more fun. I loved tasting the dough, licking the bowl and eating the warm cookies out of the oven before anyone else got one. I loved not being limited regarding how many I could have.

Even if I only came for a weekend, we always made cookies. One day, when I was eight, I was watching Grandma measure the ingredients. She would let me stir for a while and even let me pour in the ingredients after she had measured them.

My favorite part was when she'd break the eggs. I liked to watch them slowly glop into the mixing bowl. Grandma kept her hen house discoveries in a crockery bowl on the counter. This day, I asked her if I could break the eggs. She told me, no because I wasn't old enough. Then she walked a few steps away to get the butter out of the refrigerator.

That was all the opening I needed. I grabbed an egg and gave it a good crack on the edge of the cabinet just as I'd seen her do a hundred other times. Mine, though, didn't stay in the shell like hers did. It ran down the side of the cabinet and on to the floor. I stared at the gooey mess.

Grandma stopped and stared, as well. Her face changed. I could tell she was angry even though I'd never seen her mad before. I wasn't sure what she would do. I knew what Mom would have done.

Grandma didn't yell. She just marched me through the dining room, into the living room, down the hall to the bathroom. She shut the door and told me to stay there until she came back. There were two problems with this plan. First, the bathroom was a long way from the kitchen. Second, I firmly believed "Ghost Boo" lived upstairs. The stairway was right off the living room and way too close to the bathroom.

The bathroom had two doors. The second was never used. It always stayed locked from the inside. I simply ran to that door and got out. My grandmother, though, took me back and somehow locked that door, as well, so I couldn't get out.

I screamed and cried until a few minutes later she let me out. I'm sure she put me there to give herself time to clean up my mess and calm down, which she did.

When she let me out, she sat me down and explained why she didn't want me to crack the egg. She said when I was old enough she'd teach me how to do it. I told her I was sorry. She gave me a hug and everything was fine. The next week, she began teaching me how to crack an egg.

The way she disciplined was a comfort. It let me know she had my back and cared about me. I longed for that type of discipline at home. I was in charge of the household before I felt old enough to be in charge of myself. I wanted some boundaries, some things I could do and couldn't do. I knew those at Grandma's. I had little idea of what they were at home until I was severely punished for violating a rule I never knew existed.

As the years progressed, Mom was labeled manic-depressive with schizophrenic tendencies. My father concentrated on taking care of her. He abdicated other things to my care until I left home for college at age 18. Thinking about boundaries for children, especially when he had grown up with few boundaries, was the least of his worries.

FOOD BROUGHT US TOGETHER

My grandparents' house was the location of most family dinners and celebrations. These were held often, once or twice a month. The food went on forever. Everyone who came brought dishes to add to the fare. For Papaw's birthday my grandmother threw a huge dinner with all extended family present. It was replete with all of the foods I had come to know and love from my relatives' repertoires of recipes. Each had their specialties: Elizabeth's hot rolls, Aunt Cora Lee's pies, Aunt Marty's perfect mashed potatoes, Mamaw's oatmeal cake, Grandma's roast and fried chicken, Aunt Betty's dumplings and Elaine's sweet potato pie. Actually, anything my family made was delicious.

We celebrated birthdays, reunions, holidays, graduations, weddings, baptisms and special honors. These were not small affairs. By far, the best part of any family gathering was the food. The food brought us together and was the centerpiece of every event.

It is no wonder, then, when I wanted to feel comfort, I would cook something my grandmother would have served. My favorite comfort food meal I remember her making often was country-fried steak, mashed potatoes and gravy, hoecake (a fried cornbread) and oatmeal cookies. Grandma always had a vegetable. My version of the meal rarely did.

When I became an adult, I cooked many batches of oatmeal cookies. If I baked three-dozen cookies by the next morning there would be none left. Others would have several each. I, however, could not stop eating them. It seemed eating was the only way I could feel comfort. I was trying to fill some kind of empty spot in my soul or spirit.

> Eating was the only way I could feel comfort. I was trying to fill some kind of empty spot in my soul.

Some things in my childhood are indelibly imprinted on my mind. I don't feel it's anyone's fault. It's just the combination of circumstances, which led to some neural pathways being formed. The major ones were: food equals comfort; sugar anesthetizes pain. For me these became the building blocks of a deadly lifestyle.

SWEET GRACE

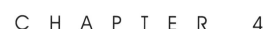

CHAPTER 4

SNAKE IN THE GRASS

"For all have sinned and fall short of the glory of God and are justified freely by His grace through the redemption that came by Christ Jesus."

Romans 3:23-24, NIV

S ummers were special because as often as I could, I stayed at Grandma and Papaw's farm. My eleventh summer was no different. Fred and Minnie (not their real names) were coming to visit. Grandma wanted to fix creek greens (a special kind of greens found near Grandma's creek) for the family dinner celebrating their arrival on Saturday evening.

She knew a special place where they were just the right size for picking. It was along the side of the dirt road near Hungry Mother Creek. She didn't share its location with everyone for fear the spot would be picked clean. Creek greens could only be harvested when they were small, otherwise they were not good.

We parked the car and walked a ways through the tall grass following a worn path. It looked like more than a few others knew Grandma's closely guarded secret.

"Grandma, I thought this spot was a secret," I said.

"This is the path folks follow to the creek for fishing. I don't think they know my secret. You have to go off the path a ways to find the patch." She continued watching carefully where she walked. "You stay right behind me. Walk where I walk."

I followed swinging the buckets we'd use to carry our finds. The sun warmed us, but a light breeze blowing across the creek moved enough air to make the day pleasant. The water gurgled as it ran over the rocks. Frogs croaked. Every once in a while I heard a splash as something jumped in the creek. If I could I would freeze the moment and take a picture to remember it exactly. Life was grand. But pictures must be taken quickly as everyone knows change can happen suddenly in Missouri.

SHE FROZE

All of a sudden, Grandma stopped, her foot frozen in the air, mid-stride. "Stop. Don't move a muscle." I became a statue. Slowly she lowered her foot to the ground behind her. In the path right in front of her lay a large light tan snake with dark brown markings. The snake seemed to stare at us with cat-like eyes. He didn't move a muscle.

My grandmother was a stalwart, farm woman who could kill a chicken, milk a cow and carry a heavy load of wet laundry up the basement stairs. Two things I knew she was afraid of—mice and snakes. The snakes around the farmhouse were much bigger and blacker than the one staring us down. The black snakes especially liked to hide in the cold, dank basement where she kept her wringer washing machine.

Every Monday, she would make sure Papaw was nearby in case the snakes showed themselves. Generally they were as scared of her as she was of them. As soon as she saw one, she ran and it ran.

This, though, was not a black snake. "What are we going to do, Grandma?" I whispered as she inched back to where I stood. The snake never moved. He held his position. He was intimidating. He just stared at us.

"We are going to very carefully inch backwards for a ways and then we turn around and hightail it out of here," she said. Her breath was coming in short bursts.

"But he's staring at us. He sees where we are going and he'll come after us."

"This kind of snake won't follow us. He's not like the black snakes that act like they're going to chase you. Really, though, the black snake is trying to get away, trying to find a place to hide. He just can't figure out which way to go and so sometimes runs towards you rather than away. Black snakes won't hurt you though."

"Why are you scared of them, then?"

She shuddered despite the warm summer sun. "I can't stand the way they come out of nowhere and scare me to death."

"What kind of snake is that one back there?" We were far enough down the grassy path that Grandma felt it safe to turn around. She nearly ran to the car. Once in the boxy Ford sedan, she sighed and gathered her breath for moment before she answered my question.

"That there was a Copperhead. Unlike the black snake, if he bites you it will hurt, a lot. It is poisonous, but people I've seen who've been bitten haven't died."

"He looked like he could eat us. I didn't like his eyes. They looked mad."

"Snakes are snakes. I don't know of any snake that mixes well with humans. I'm glad you are okay. I couldn't forgive myself if anything happened to you. With a child, a Copperhead's bite could be very dangerous."

I scooted over close to her in the seat and lay my head on her shoulder. "Nothing could ever happen to me when I'm with you," I said with unmitigated devotion. "I love you, Grandma."

"Oh child, if you loved me half as much as I love you, it'd be enough."

GOOD GUYS AND BAD GUYS

To me there are two kinds of men in the world—black snakes and Copperheads. The first kind of men I knew well and until the age of 11, I figured these were the only kind of men in the world. These are the good guys, the quiet super-heroes.

They are the ordinary, every day variety you might find in a basement washroom. They do their job of killing rodents. They don't bite. They don't want credit. They just want to be left alone and if not, they will scurry out of the way.

All of the men I had known had been good guys—my great-grandfather, my grandfather and father were all loving, family men and active Christians. They were committed and loyal to their beliefs, not prone to being loud, obnoxious, angry or forceful. They were pleasant, caring and concerned. They never yelled. They were quiet, gentle giants of faith. I trusted them completely.

Unfortunately, there are also bad guys, the Copperheads. The Copperhead does have some distinctive differences from the black snake. They can bite and their bite is poisonous. It may not kill, but the person bitten can be scarred for life.

Up until age 11, I had known a couple of Copperheads who were boys, not men. Both of them wanted me to play patient to their version of doctor. I hadn't put a name on them at that time, but they definitely were Copperheads in the making.

The worst Copperhead was Fred, the friend the entire family loved. Fred was loud, selfish and needy. The day he and his wife, Minnie, were scheduled to arrive, we were gathered at Grandma's and Papaw's. The men sat under the shade tree. The kids played hide and seek. The women cooked in the kitchen.

THEY'RE HERE

My brother saw them first. His yells of, "They're here," were drowned out by the noise of the car engine pulling into the driveway. Grandma literally leaped out the back door and ran to the car, beating everyone else who watched her in awe. She threw open the car door and gave Minnie a bear hug I was sure would crush her. It had been a year since they had seen each other.

"Where are my hugs and kisses?" Fred stepped around from the driver's side. He wore a crisp white shirt open at the throat, long sleeves rolled up and gray creased trousers. A cigar hung from his mouth, which he removed, threw in the driveway and crushed beneath his black dress shoes.

The little girls ran into his open arms. Most everyone loved Fred. Making his way to a chair under the shade tree, Fred sat down. "OK, who's first?"

"Me. Me." The younger girls jostled each other out of the way to be the first in line.

It was a little like the kissing booth at the fair. We knew the drill. Sit on his lap, give him a kiss and he'd pull a silver dollar out of one of our ears. He pulled silver dollars out of the boys' ears, too, but they didn't have to give him kisses. He just performed the trick. They would get tired of it after one time and go tease the cats in the barn. The girls got as many chances as there were silver dollars. He seemed to have an endless supply.

The year before I had 10 silver dollars, which I used to help buy my first full-size bike. It almost seemed like ill-gotten gain. I never liked Fred's kisses. His mouth was all lip and tasted like cigars. I much preferred the sweet peck on the cheek Papaw gave. I seemed to be the only girl reluctant to give more than one kiss, but then I was the oldest.

The Saturday evening dinner included creek greens seasoned with bacon fat (Grandma had sent her hired man back to gather them), homemade rolls, fried chicken, mashed potatoes, fried apples, three kinds of pie and oatmeal cookies. After supper was over and the dishes washed, the adults sat in the lawn chairs in the side yard overlooking the road while the children caught fireflies. Fred's cigar smoke added a different atmosphere to the clean country air that existed in Papaw's yard.

I had been staying for a few weeks with my grandparents. That evening everyone headed home, but I stayed. My parents would be coming back the next day after church for the seining (dragging a seine net through the pond to catch fish) and fish fry. They said I could stay Saturday. On Sunday I could leave or stay the rest of the week. Mom preferred I come home to help her. I preferred Grandma's house.

UPSTAIRS

My grandparents' white two-story farmhouse had three bedrooms upstairs and one downstairs. Grandma and Papaw slept downstairs. When I spent the night I would either sleep on a pallet beside my grandmother or on the living room couch because I was afraid of "Boo," the ghost from our stories. She explained because Minnie and Fred would be down the hall, I shouldn't be scared. I could sleep upstairs.

At bedtime, I reluctantly went upstairs to the first room at the top of the stairway. It was closer to the stairs and, therefore, made me feel closer to my grandparents. Their room was directly below.

The windows were open to the summer breeze. I could hear the rumbling of Papaw and Grandma's voices as they talked before going to sleep. I heard Papaw pray with her as he did every night. Then, I heard their soft snores. It was a security I loved. I fell sound asleep.

The next morning, Minnie went downstairs early to help Grandma fix breakfast and get ready for the fish fry later that day.

Yesterday when Fred asked me to sit on his lap and give him a kiss, his hands seemed to stray accidently. I ignored it, got up quickly and left thinking I must have been mistaken. Those kinds of imaginary acts happened often when Fred was around. I was keenly aware I was developing quicker than most of the girls in my class. I was the first of the girls I knew to reach puberty.

COPPERHEAD IN MY ROOM

That morning, though, imagination played no part. As I lay asleep, Fred tiptoed into the room. I woke when I heard the door open. I saw him come in. I quickly shut my eyes and pretended to sleep. In my mind, I fervently prayed for God to intervene. But Fred was still there.

"Wake up, Little Darling. Come on, time to get up and give your old Fred a kiss." He leaned his entire body over the bed and gave me a kiss I was sure would bruise my lips. I still pretended to sleep.

He jerked back the sheet. I could feel the morning breeze on my skin. I was well aware my short nightgown covered very little. "Come on now. I know you're awake."

My mind went to the incident by the creek. When the Copperhead appeared, Grandma froze. I became a statue. Inside, though, I prayed, "Help me, Jesus. Help me, Jesus. Help me, Jesus." I played dead.

Every second of the next few minutes is etched indelibly in my mind. His hands were all over me. I attempted to go elsewhere in my mind to think good thoughts, but it wasn't working. I prayed for God to send Grandma or Minnie up the stairs.

Instead Fred began touching me in places my mother had said boys should not touch me until I was married. The touching felt painful. I willed the tears away. Frozen in time and space my mind went numb; my body limp. I prayed as never before. Again, I begged God to intervene.

I was afraid what Fred might do. I couldn't move. I couldn't breathe. I was mortified by his actions and I was sure it wouldn't be long before something very bad would happen. In sheer desperation, I sent up a final, silent prayer. It was much simpler this time. "Help, God. Help."

When no lightening bolt appeared, a million thoughts crossed my mind about how I could stop what appeared to be the inevitable. I could claw his face. I could kick him. I could scream at the top of my lungs. I saw the actions in my mind, but could not make my body move.

Then I heard the answer to my prayer.

"Fred, time for breakfast." It was Minnie's voice calling from the bottom of the stairway just outside the room.

"Be right down, Sugar." Fred called back.

He leaned close and said gruffly in my ear, "Open your eyes." He smelled of cigar smoke. I disobeyed. My eyes stayed shut. I didn't move.

Before I knew it, I heard the door close. He had left without doing what I feared. Several seconds passed. It felt like an eternity. The stairs creaked as he descended.

I sucked in a big breath of air, but lay still. I was afraid to open my eyes. I could only assume he had feared his wife would come and find him if he didn't go downstairs. But would he eat and come back? I opened my eyes and forced myself to dress quickly.

WHO COULD I TELL?

I ran downstairs to the bathroom. Laughter came from the kitchen. How could he laugh with them after what he did?

I wanted to take a bath, but Grandma would think it odd. I took one last night. No one took a bath every day on the farm. Water from a well, especially in the summer, tended to be scarce. I washed myself as best I could trying to wash the places he touched. I brushed my teeth and straightened my hair. I wandered into the kitchen and sat down in my usual spot between Grandma and Papaw.

"Good morning, Sleepyhead." Grandma laughed. "Let me get you some bacon, eggs and toast. You want juice?"

"Yes, and some strawberry preserves for the toast. Maybe two pieces of toast." I felt empty and slightly nauseous. Maybe food would do the trick.

I ate my breakfast as quickly as my stomach could handle and then asked if I could go change into my dress. Grandma cocked her head and raised her eyebrows. Most of the time, I stayed with her in the kitchen until the last minute possible.

I pondered telling her, but I couldn't. Fred was Minnie's husband. Grandma and Minnie were best friends. Did Minnie know? Did she know what her good church-going husband was trying to do with me? Did she know what he would do if he had another chance? Would she be mad? Would she blame me? Would she believe me? It would break Grandma's heart to know what Minnie's husband was like.

Mom taught me adults were always right. I couldn't bear to think Grandma might not believe me. They would think I was trying to accuse Fred falsely. They would think me a troublemaker. It would make Grandma so sad. No, I couldn't risk telling anyone. Of course, I couldn't tell Mom. Everyone knew she was not well. It might make her worse.

> Would she blame me? Would she believe me? I couldn't risk telling anyone.

Upstairs I dressed in record time, packed my clothes and took my bag downstairs. For an 11-year old who had been in charge of a household, I figured I would have to protect myself. I vowed not to stay overnight at Grandma's while Fred and Minnie were there. I would stay away from Fred as much as I could when I was at an event where he was.

Mom was surprised when I put my suitcase in the car the minute they drove up. "You coming home with us?"

"Yeah, I think Grandma and Minnie have lots of catching up to do. They don't need me underfoot."

"I could really use your help," she said. "Next week everyone's coming to our house for country ham and red-eye gravy." When it was time to go, Fred kissed Mom, pulled a quarter out of Renee's ear for a kiss and then wanted to do the same thing for me.

"We have to go." I ran to the car.

"Come back here and give Fred a kiss." Mom stood with her hands on her hips.

I couldn't figure a quick way out of it, so I came back and allowed a kiss. It seemed he held it longer than usual. When I tried to pull away he held my chin, looked me in the eyes and grinned in a way that made me shudder. Renee only got a quarter for her kiss, but I got a silver dollar. When I got in the car, she complained. I gave her my silver dollar. "Thank you, Sissy," she said her eyes beaming.

She was too young to understand. I couldn't have held the coin a minute longer without letting out a blood-curdling scream. I could tell no one what it represented. He couldn't force me to keep the money. I knew he gave it to me to let me know there were more if there was more forthcoming from me. I wanted nothing more from him, ever.

I tried to approach my aunt the next weekend at Grandma's house. I caught her alone. "You ever think it unusual that Fred only kisses the girls?"

"Well, I think it would be unusual if he kissed the boys."

"Your girls ever said anything about him like they were afraid of him?"

"Everyone loves Fred."

"You ever afraid of him?"

"Why, no. Never." She walked away presumably to help get food on the table. I expected her to ask why I was asking, but she didn't. From that one overture, I figured I was the only one Fred attempted this with. Fred didn't bother me anymore after that summer. Although they came for a few more visits, they only stayed a few days or so at a time.

DENIAL

I never told anyone what Fred did to me that summer until I met my husband. Before we got married I told him what happened and that it might be difficult for me on the wedding night. What I thought would be difficult he overcame with tenderness and caring.

In my 30s, I decided I had held the secret long enough. One day I told Mom what Fred had done and why I was always scared of him. By this time, he had already passed away.

"That's a lie." Her green eyes flashed a dark color. "That never happened."

"It did happen."

"No, it didn't and don't ever say another thing like that to me again."

"Did he ever do anything to you?"

"This is my house and you are not to talk about this again. Do you hear me?"

"It happened, Mom."

"You are making it up."

"I'm not a little kid, Mom. I know what happened."

"It did not happen. You are lying."

"I would not make up something like that. Why would I?"

She walked out of the room. I never talked with her about it again.

I tried to entrust my mother with my secret. It seems it was a secret she decided to keep from herself.

Years later, in a class I began to learn more about adult men who molest young girls. For one thing most pedophiles don't molest just one child, but many. They choose those who are vulnerable. For years, I felt what he did to me must have been my fault, not his. My blossoming body must have caused him to be led astray.

Although I cannot and will not blame my weight gain on Fred, I do know that from that time on, I was scared of men who acted like Copperheads. Other pre-teen and teenage girls I ran around with wanted to be as attractive as possible to guys. In many situations young men tended to take after Fred more than the wonderful role models I had in my father and grandfathers. Those role models made me want to keep trying to find the right man, one of the good guys who respected me and loved me for myself.

One thing I felt fairly early in my encounter with bad guys is good guys are no match for bad guys. Black snakes run away and prefer not to enter a conflict.

As a kid all I knew was Copperheads stand their ground. If I was going to be protected, I was going to have to come up with a plan to do it myself just like I did with Fred. This plan had to be all encompassing, something that would keep the bad guys away.

Fat, lots and lots of fat, is the best deterrent I know for bad guys. And if they come after me, I can always sit on them.

I can protect myself. I don't need any help from anyone else.

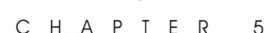

CHAPTER 5

NO BOUNDARIES

*"Like a city whose walls are broken through
is a person who lacks self-control."*

Proverbs 25:28, NIV

E very day of high school revolved around one question, "Do you want to go to King's for lunch?" We could go off campus to fast food places. King's was right across the road from my high school. It had booths so we could cram in as many friends as possible. Each booth had speakers where we placed our order. Outside was the drive-in where those in vehicles could do the same thing. It was the happening place to be during the day, as well as nights and weekends.

The best thing about King's for me, though, was the Cheese Frenchee. This was a grilled cheese sandwich on steroids. Made with Texas toast and thick slices of Velveeta cheese, it was a breaded and deep-fried delicacy.

Mom gave me money for school lunch each week. However, no self-respecting high school junior would dare eat a school lunch unless, of course, it was snowing or raining. The sandwich I loved, worshipped really, cost three times the price of school lunch.

I had a job after school two hours a day and on Saturdays for about five hours. I got paid minimum wage for 15 hours. Out of that I had to pay for gas in my car, any clothes I bought and anything extra I wanted for lunches.

My pay didn't stretch far enough for me to eat a Cheese Frenchee every day and save money for college. I really did want to go to college. I knew I could get scholarships, but I would have to have spending money while there. Mom told me this had to come from the money I earned from my part-time job.

That didn't matter. Every day I'd sit in class and dream of Cheese Frenchees. One of my first visions was of a Cheese Frenchee. I guess it wasn't a vision per se, however it was something I could see in my mind and almost taste. It certainly set me on a mission to try and do everything I could to eat one every day for lunch.

Besides funds, another issue with going to King's every day was getting served and getting back to class on time. If I could cut the hour before lunch or the hour after lunch we could make it. The hour before lunch was nearly impossible. The teacher was a stickler about attendance records. However, the teacher for typing, my class after lunch, didn't take attendance. I had never cut a class, but this class was boring. I fell asleep a lot. Everything was in the book and all we did was practice during class. I decided I'd practice at King's or during study hall. The call of the Cheese Frenchee was louder than the click of the typewriter keys. The problem, though, was in-class quizzes. I caught a few classes and few quizzes, but when I got my mid-term grade report I knew I was in trouble.

NEWSPAPER VISION

It was important to me to make good grades because I wanted to go to a private Christian university and major in journalism. I wanted to start an inter-denominational Christian newspaper funded entirely from advertising revenue. In the 1970s, the only Christian newspapers were denominational newspapers with one point of view. I felt God had shown me a different newspaper, which told the good news about what God was doing in and through His people, various churches and different programs. I wanted to know how to write, edit and publish such a publication. I knew one day I would be part of it.

The vision drove my desire to make good grades to get the scholarships. I had already taken the ACT and made application to Oklahoma Baptist University (OBU). My goal was clear. My desire set. I was a walled city, but there was a breach in the wall. It was the size of a triangular piece of Cheese Frenchee.

I needed to go to typing class so I turned my sights towards the class before lunch. I decided to see if I could work my wiles on the office secretary. She knew and trusted me. All I had to do was wave at her as I passed by the office and she'd take me off the roll. I began trying it when I left early for lunch, sticking my head in one day I told her that I had to check the school newspaper proof at the printer's and class was just review.

From then on, I just waved when coming or going and she marked me off the list. It worked marvelously until the teacher found out I hadn't gotten detention for my tardies. I wasn't getting unexcused absences. She caught me after one of the rare classes where I'd been present and let me know I needed to be in class.

"The next test scores are going to be significantly lower for those who are absent for any reason," she said. The way she looked at me, I knew she was telling the truth. I could see the army of Cheese Frenchees slipping away from me. What could I do? I had to pass this class, as well.

I was not a veteran at skipping class. This was the first year I had ever tried it. The call of the Cheese Frenchee, though, was all consuming. I had another friend who also had a sixth hour study hall. Since I had a standing excuse to get out of that period, we began going to King's right after fifth hour. I'd grab a sandwich at lunch as well, but I still had my Cheese Frenchee. I had enough to buy one every day if I babysat as well as working my part-time job, but I wasn't saving any money for college.

It seemed logical to me to find a way to eat what I wanted, what I craved.

It seemed logical to me, for some reason, to find a way to eat what I wanted, what I craved. The thought never occurred that a harmless sandwich could be responsible for adding additional weight. Before I knew it, I had gained 40 pounds.

The incongruous thing is I so wanted to look like the cheerleaders and pom pom girls who jumped around at football and basketball games. They were the smart, popular girls. A lot of them were in my honors English class. I knew them, but I didn't run in their crowd.

I couldn't eat Cheese Frenchees and lose weight. But the Cheese Frenchee won out every time. I can't go back and get inside my 16-year-old brain. I wanted to save money for college and make good grades. I felt I knew what God wanted me to do with my life. I had a purpose to head toward. Why would I allow something as ridiculous as the desire for a sandwich to have the possibility of ruining my grades and a scholarship? The desire to save money for college and make good grades was out of sync with the desire to skip class and eat a grilled cheese sandwich, no matter how spectacular.

CHEESE FRENCHEE LAND

High school was a stressful time. There was the desire to fit in, the desire to be popular, the desire to go to college and the desire to get a degree in order to get a job and not live under my mother's roof for the rest of my life.

A Cheese Frenchee provided an oasis in the middle of a difficult day. I would do almost anything to bite into that delicious sandwich. It would carry me away into a land where for 30 minutes to an hour, I could bask in the aromas, the tastes, and the feels of food filling me completely.

In Cheese Frenchee land, I wasn't an unpopular high school girl; I was a calm, cool and collected woman who was in control of her situation. It didn't matter if others didn't deem me popular, I had Mr. Frenchee. He was enough for me.

Because I was working and had a little money, I had the ability to obtain what I wanted to eat. This felt like I was controlling my life. No one was telling me what I could and could not eat. No one was punishing me for snagging candy from the kitchen or eating an extra cookie. No one was dictating what I did with my body. It was all me. If I gained weight, it was all right because I was in control of my destiny. What I wanted in the moment trumped any long-term benefit of not indulging.

WEIGHT ON MY MIND

I really cannot remember a time when I didn't either want to lose weight, was trying to lose weight or thinking of a way to lose weight. It was constantly on my mind even while growing up. In grade school, I felt like a big blob next to the other girls in my class. Looking back at my pictures, I don't really look fat. Still I distinctly remember being larger than others in my classroom.

I can remember Mom and Grandma telling me I needed to lose weight. This would happen every time I outgrew clothes. As the oldest child and grandchild, there were no hand-me-downs. I had to have new clothes. Maybe that was the reason they encouraged me to lose weight.

I seemed to have masked my issues whatever they were. I told myself I was just a little larger than everyone else. I told myself I didn't want a boyfriend. I told myself I didn't need to be a size 10. Actually, I don't ever remember being a size 10. I remember being husky girl's sizes and then, a size 12 women's. There were no in-betweens. I felt out of place with my world.

My thinking process tended to begin in a general feeling of malaise and would spiral down to a pinpointed angst, which always needed to be assuaged with food. Food ceased to become a necessary source of fuel; it was my life. I did not eat to live, I lived to eat and as much as I could, any time I could.

PAIN ANESTHETIZED

Whatever happened I would go to food to anesthetize the pain. A teacher criticized me in front of the class. That's all right, only another class hour before I can get to the Cheese Frenchee. The popular girls laughed when I walked by in my last year's madras plaid jacket? Only three more hours to King's. I needed a bigger size in jeans? That's okay; I can go out with my friends and get food. Pizza will do the trick this time. It doesn't really matter. It just needs to have bread, cheese and lots of grease; it needs to fill the void inside.

> Whatever happened I would go to food to anesthetize the pain.

If anyone had asked me the question, who's in control of your life? I would have answered God, of course. It was a stock answer, but not real in any sense. I knew God, but He wasn't in control. Food was in control.

A theme had formed. I allowed my physical body to dictate decisions rather than my soul or spirit. The Bible says the deeds of the flesh are bad,[1] right? I have to squelch evil desires. I did squelch most of them. I didn't drink. I didn't smoke pot or do drugs like many of my friends did. I wasn't sexually promiscuous. I didn't go to wild parties. And yet, there was this emptiness. I filled it with food because that was acceptable.

Going out to eat, talking and laughing, was a fun way to spend an evening. It was not a sin. The difficulty was that I used food in a different way than most.

In the times I was not with people, my soul cried out for attention, for comfort, for significance, for love, for relationship, for acceptance. I didn't know how to fill those needs with anything except food, preferably something sweet or something with lots of bread. No one I knew saw overeating as satisfying a desire of the flesh. It was acceptable in the church. People must eat.

I had never been taught how to fill my inner longings. If anyone had asked me what he or she could do to help me, I would not know what to say. I certainly didn't know what to tell myself. I didn't even realize I was filling emotional needs with food.

I hadn't processed through the fact I was spending all my money on food and would have to get a job in college just to buy tuna fish and chicken noodle soup. Sacrificing my immediate wants for a long-term goal was a concept I knew in theory, but couldn't put into practice.

Sadly, my city had no walls.[2] I had no boundaries where food was concerned. Already I had come to rely on its constant presence and unrelenting ability to fix whatever ailed me.

ENDNOTES

1. Galatians 5:19-21, NIV

2. Proverbs 25:28, NIV

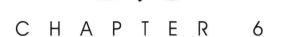

C H A P T E R 6

EATING CAN BE PAINFUL

"Trust God from the bottom of your heart; don't try to figure out everything on your own. Listen for God's voice in everything you do, everywhere you go; He's the One who will keep you on track. Don't assume that you know it all. Run to God. Run from evil. Your body will glow with health, your very bones will vibrate with life."

Proverbs 3:5-8, MSG

W e were embarking on a grand adventure. My high school friend and I had both graduated from college. We were moving to Virginia.

Once I graduated college, my mother was adamant I should not live at home. This ultimatum was born of the fact she had taken on the role a mom should assume with my brother and sister. She had been touched by God and was on her road to healing. I admired her growing strength of character. I knew she was telling me I could not come back home because she was in the role of the mom now. If I came back it would usurp her rightful authority. Her matter of fact statement came at me: "You will not be living with us after you graduate college."

My senior year in college I was constantly afraid and anxious. The standard question of what are you going to do when you graduate was very intimidating. I had no idea. I wanted to use my journalism/religion major in writing and publications.

I had the vision firmly in place. It had driven me to pursue a degree combination that didn't exist at the time. I created it from a loophole called the "interdisciplinary major." I believed the newspaper I wanted to publish would one day exist. Regional Christian newspapers were already cropping up in major cities, but I hadn't really heard about them. I only knew the desire God had placed in my heart and gathered the education necessary.

GRADUATE, THEN WHAT?

To begin with, I would have to take a different kind of position to gain some experience before the job I had envisioned came along. Prior to graduation I had interviewed with the Southern Baptist Foreign Mission Board (FMB) for a job as a press writer. The job was writing news stories based on interviews with missionaries who came home on furlough or sent in information from the field. The office was in Richmond, Virginia, 900 miles from my hometown. I thought I had the job.

The man who flew down to OBU to interview me was a graduate of my university. I had a good interview. Now when people asked what I was going to do when I graduated, I had an answer. Then I got the letter; the one that said they had hired someone else. I was crushed. I went with my back-up plan of working for the summer as arts and crafts director at Camp Soaring Hawk in southern Missouri. I also had charge over five spoiled girls. We bonded, though, and by July I came to care about them and they about me.

Our families weren't supposed to call camp unless it was an emergency. When I was told I had a phone call I was apprehensive someone was hurt or sick. I ran to the phone. It was my Dad. Now I was sure something was up with Mom.

"Don't worry everyone is fine," he said. "I wanted to call to tell you we got a letter today from the FMB. Do you want me to send it to you or open it and read it to you?"

"What are you waiting for Dad? Open it."

"It says they want you in Richmond in August to start the job as press writer. The supervisor would like you to call him at your earliest convenience."

I whooped and hollered. I was so excited. I would have to leave camp early. Actually, I left the next week to pack and get ready for the trip across the United States. I had a mixture of excitement and dread.

MOVING

On a whim I wrote my friend, Jacque, and I asked if she wanted to come with me, help me drive and have an adventure into the unknown. She jumped at the chance. She wanted to work as a restaurant manager and felt Virginia might be the place.

I had a 1968 Dodge Rambler my pastor had sold me the year before. He promised me it was in great shape. One advantage was the Rambler was roomy. We crammed it full of most of what we thought we needed, mainly clothes, a few kitchen items and bedding.

We figured we'd get a furnished apartment. We had lots of those in our college town. When we got to Richmond they seemed non-existent. Even the concept was foreign to most people. We loved the temporary quarters the FMB provided, but we had a date by which we had to leave as furloughing missionaries were due to arrive and needed the apartment.

Desperate to find a place, we shared it as a prayer request at the young adult Bible study group. A young woman came up to us afterwards and told us about a place. An elderly lady was in a nursing home and her family wanted to rent out the bottom floor of her house with all furniture included. It had two bedrooms, bath, kitchen, dining room, and living room with fireplace and laundry. It was less rent than most apartments back home.

It was on West Ladies Mile Road. Unless it was falling apart or in a seedy neighborhood, we knew we'd take it and we did. It was a quaint, story and a half brick with off-white trim. A brick walkway led to the front door. The driveway led to the back where an off-white wood fence enclosed a picturesque yard. Azalea bushes dotted the landscape. The gate opened to a brick patio and glassed in back porch. Off the back porch was the kitchen with glass doors and antique dishes. It was fully stocked with pots and pans, dishtowels, potholders and silverware.

I chose the bedroom with dark wood furniture. The four-poster bed had a large carved headboard. Everything matched. It was like something out of a movie setting. The living room had a Queen Anne style sofa and chairs and a wood-burning fireplace. The dining room was set with everything we needed.

It was beyond anything we could have thought of, asked for or imagined.[1] The woman's niece lived in the upstairs apartment, so if we had problems we could talk to her. For the most part, she stayed to herself. The house was perfect. We were immediately accepted as tenants because of the reputation of my employer.

NEW JOB

At the job I was writing all day, which I loved. I wrote everything on an electric typewriter, which was the computer of the day with no spell check. Writing about missionaries, along with their work and their successes, was thrilling.

A veteran foreign missionary was the executive director. We had the privilege of hearing him speak in chapel once a week. He was a master encourager, always talking about how those working at the FMB were holding the rope for those toiling overseas. He emphasized that one department or job was not any more important than another. Janitors, secretaries, press writers and regional directors were all equally important in helping maintain the welfare of the missionaries. I loved being a part of a group whose main focus, whether vacuuming the floor or typing a press release, was for the greater good of mankind.

I became the staff writer for Latin America. I wrote stories and chose pictures to release with the articles out of the hundreds missionaries sent. Yet I still have never traveled to any part of Latin America.

The position required a lot from me. It was sometimes overwhelming. As writers, we had to check and double-check facts in the information missionaries sent to us mostly via cassette tapes. We had to be sensitive to political issues within countries making sure we didn't put missionaries in danger.

Some of the stories ended up in press releases and others in full-length stories sent to various denominational magazines.

In 1976, a major earthquake in Guatemala had my area of the world hopping to provide disaster relief. I was writing several stories a day and combing through thousands of pictures to find the one or two to illustrate the depth of the story. I loved the fast pace and excitement of writing about an ever-changing world. It was fulfilling and exhilarating at the same time.

With this, though, I felt a self-inflicted pressure to perform perfectly. The other young woman who had been hired at the same time was from Texas. She was a brilliant scholar who had been at the top of her graduating class. She rarely made mistakes. Her copy was always clean and crisp.

> I felt a self-inflicted pressure to perform perfectly.

Eating became difficult during this time in my life. I seemed to be constantly on the run trying to manage my life and participate in everything I could. I ate whatever I wanted, whenever I wanted. I tried to keep a handle on things to some degree. By that I mean I ate a salad every once in awhile.

TREE

To my new friends I was "Tree." I had never really had a nickname before, but I loved the newness of it. Part of the nickname came from shortening my name, but the other aspect was my fascination with the huge, old trees on the east coast. I was constantly saying, "Missouri does not have trees like this." My new friends thought my intrigue with what they saw as ordinary, very strange.

Majestic trees are some of my favorite things. They seem to touch heaven with their height. Lying on the ground and looking up, all I could see was the tops of the trees reaching always upwards. I loved going to the Blue Ridge Mountains to see the trees. In the mountains the trees really do reach heaven. The environment touches a deep part of my soul that makes me sigh and relax; all cares and worries relieved.

That's why I was excited to go on a camping trip with my friends. We were looking forward to a weekend away from work and distractions in order to have a great time in the outdoors and with each other.

We loaded the van with all the gear and headed out. It was a little nippy for spring, but we were prepared with coats and sleeping bags. We were planning to hike a while on Saturday after camping Friday night. We set up our tents, built a campfire, roasted hot dogs and marshmallows, made s'mores, sang songs, told stories and then went to bed. Already it had been a great time.

The next morning was to be the hike. I woke refreshed, but with some pain in my abdomen. As the morning progressed, the pain got worse. We broke camp and packed up. We planned to drive to a spot on the hiking trail that afforded some of the most spectacular views.

My friends were worried. I told them to go ahead. I knew enough to know it wasn't an appendicitis attack. It only hurt when I sat or stood. The only position where I could get any kind of relief was curled up in a ball in the back seat. I took an acetaminophen and tried to rest. From time-to-time I would sit up to see if it was any better. It wasn't.

They cut their hike short and took me home. The pain was still bad, but began to subside a little as long as I could lie down. I felt better Sunday, but the pain came back Sunday night. I called the doctor first thing on Monday.

STRESS?

At the doctor's office, they had me drink white, chalky stuff in order to get an x-ray of my colon. When the doctor showed me the x-ray, it looked as if a giant had taken my colon and squeezed it in different places. He explained I had something called Irritable Bowel Syndrome.

"Are you under a lot of stress?" he asked.

I thought about my answer. I was working in my first full-time job. I knew I had not been the first pick for the job. I felt I had to work extra hard to prove myself. Every time I made a mistake, I was sure my boss was asking himself, "Tell me again why I hired her."

My boss only pointed out my errors so I could learn from my mistakes. If I made the same error again, he pointed it out again, so I would learn again. I put way too much pressure on myself. My boss did not expect perfection, but I did.

I was the leader of our young adult Bible study, which had now grown to over 50 people. I was responsible for planning and leading the Bible study, organizing fellowships and making sure everything went smoothly. We met weekly. I loved leading, but I felt I had to have everything lined out in impeccable order.

I was over two days drive away from my Midwest home. I couldn't just drop in for a visit. I only had one week vacation a year which was spent coming home at Christmas. This was different from college where I could come home for anything and everything including holidays and birthdays.

The small things that everyone takes for granted such as paying monthly bills, keeping a budget and keeping everything nice in the beautiful house full of antique furniture, was taking a toll on me.

Yes, I realized, I was stressed.

My whole body was exhausted—my spirit, my mind, my emotions, my physical body. I was helpless and weak. Things inside of me weren't fitting together. I was pulled in so many different directions.

I loved everything I was doing, which included work, Bible study, meetings, planning, chorale, fellowship times and helping at the mission center. It was constant activity. Not only that, but I had started what would become another theme in my life. I wasn't just involved in being a part of things; I pretty much led whatever I was involved in.

I was feeling overwhelmed. It was like part of me had fallen and couldn't get up. I pushed myself because I thought I had to lead. Surely this was what God wanted me to do. By doing what He wanted me to do I would make Him happy. If He was happy with me, I would earn His favor. When the stress got to me, I ate.

I knew I needed discipline to just be quiet before God and commune with Him, but somehow all the doing was crowding that out. I prayed, "When nothing else seems to fit together, when all my strength is gone, You are my strength, Lord. Teach me my limitations."

I'm sure God was talking to me about my limitations way before things got to this point. I just wasn't listening until I my body began feeling the symptoms of stress. To this day, I don't think I've ever experienced such a horrific pain, except when I've had surgeries. It shut down my entire body.

IRRITABLE BOWEL SYNDROME

I looked at the doctor and said, "I never thought of it as stress, but I guess it is."

He explained stress affects people in different ways. Stress was affecting me by clenching my colon to the point the pain became debilitating.

"So it's not psychosomatic?" I asked. I was always concerned about emotional illness.

"No, it's real. There are some things we can do about it."

He gave me a muscle relaxer to take when the pain got too severe. In addition he gave me a diet to follow. Mainly, I was to cut out sugar, fats, most grains and salads and raw vegetables. I heard the words, "cut out .... salads and raw vegetables." I never liked them anyway. That was easy.

For the first time, a doctor talked to me about losing weight and following a diet. I did follow part of the diet. I didn't eat salad or raw vegetables. I also attempted eating broiled or baked chicken and meats. I continued eating sugar and grains, though.

I hated the muscle relaxer because it knocked me out. Whatever event I was trying to make sure I could attend was still not possible because I was sleeping instead of hurting. I had a talk with myself about this problem. "If stress goes to your colon, you just need to not have stress. Just give it to God and stop worrying about everything being done to perfection."

I also gave up some responsibilities and invited another member of the young adult group to be co-director. We began rotating responsibility for weekly sessions. I was starting to realize why they called working 40 hours a week full-time. There was not much else I could do besides work, but I continued to try.

SAVING THE WORLD

Jacque tried to talk some sense into me. One day she said, "You can't save the whole world by yourself."

I answered, "Yes, but I can try." That was my mindset. The weight of the world was on my shoulders. I had to hold up my corner or it would topple off its axis.

The disposition towards colon issues runs in my family, so I did not take the diagnosis lightly. However, I had brushed over some important areas the doctor mentioned, mainly cutting out sugar, greasy foods and grains.

Donuts and fried cinnamon rolls were becoming my every day go-to food. I justified them as necessary to ease my stress. Even though the doctor said these kinds of foods could cause distress, they didn't. As the comfort foods I'd come to know and love, they seemed to work to relieve the anxiety of being everything to everybody. I didn't want the searing pain in my abdomen, but I wanted to keep doing what I was doing.

Food also made social gatherings more fun. The young adults in my group did not drink alcohol, but we made up for it with food. We'd have meals at each other's houses, delicious sugary snacks during fellowship each week and church carry-in meals. As a single woman, these were important times to connect with others.

From time to time, I vowed to get my life in order. I confessed not doing it. I asked for forgiveness for not following what I knew were basic things I needed to be doing such as eating healthy food and disciplining my body, thoughts, emotions, attitudes and desires.

I was going so fast doing things that I had not taken time to be in God's presence. I was trying to figure everything out on my own like I had done all my life. Instead, I needed to lean on Him and listen to His voice. I needed to fully rely on Him. I figured I knew it all. I was not turning to God. I was turning to food to keep me from falling completely apart and, as a result, I was gaining weight. I might have sidetracked my IBS, but now I had a much bigger problem.

I was trying to figure everything out on my own.

None of my clothes fit. I was buying clothes for work in a size larger than what I had. I had outgrown everything I had brought with me. I was the largest young woman in our office, but not overwhelmingly huge in my way of thinking.

GLOWING?

I knew God's promises and loved the one in Proverbs 3:5-8 that said if I would trust God and run to Him instead of trying to figure everything out on my own, my body would glow with health and my very bones would vibrate with life.[2]

I wasn't glowing, though. I felt like a tarnished copper kettle, corroded, grimy and sooty. I wanted God to just take a cloth, polish and clean me like new. I told Him I was tired, hungry, lonely, angry, confused and overwhelmed, and if He would just show me what to do I'd cooperate and follow instructions.

He was telling me to come to Him and He'd lead me, but that meant more time in Bible study and prayer. I just wanted one of those genie-in-a-bottle magic cures. I wanted God to grant my wish and put my life in order. I'd go to sleep one night and I'd wake up feeling healthy the next morning.

It would not be the first time I asked for such a miracle. I had little concept of the fact that as a Christian I had been given the greatest miracle of all when I accepted Christ. The Holy Spirit was placed inside me and was ready to help me clean up my life. I was telling Him to do it Himself.

Unfortunately, or fortunately, however you want to look at it, He doesn't work that way.

ENDNOTES

1. Ephesians 3:20, NIV
2. Proverbs 3:5-8, MSG

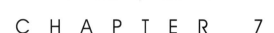

CHAPTER 7

TIME TO GROW UP

*"When I was a child, I talked like a child, I spoke
and thought and reasoned as a child. But when
I grew up, I put away childish things."*

1 Corinthians 13:11, NLT

M y boyfriend, Roy, and I had broken up before I went
to Virginia. Even though I loved him, I was sure the
relationship was over. We had remained friends and
within a year, I got a long letter from him. He was not a letter
writer. This four-page letter described everything he was
doing, thinking and feeling.

Because of his personality, I knew the letter meant we would
never speak to each other again or we would get married. I
wasn't sure what to write back. Then I got another letter asking
if he could see me over Thanksgiving. I wasn't coming home
then, but I gave him my schedule for Christmas.

We saw each other every day during Christmas break. He
asked me to marry him at midnight the day after Christmas.
We were sitting at a booth in the Interstate Pancake House.

He simply said, "I don't want to be apart from you. I think we should get married." I agreed. We sealed it in prayer.

Nearly four years after I met Roy, I became his bride. I felt I could never possibly love him any more than I did that day. I had lived a fairly selfish life, thinking only of my future, my work, my writing, my ministry, my friends. Now there was another person in the mix I loved dearly and who loved me. I never wanted to be apart from him. We promised to grow old together. We would both need to learn how to do that.

Although our story has a positive outcome, 36 years and counting, there was a time when it almost came to a screeching halt. In every way, the fault was mine. I had a love affair, not with another man, but with food.

EATING NORMALLY

Soon after we got married, Roy said to me, "I love the way you look, but please don't gain any more weight." This was a heart-felt concern of his. He is tall and normal weight and never overeats. He sometimes eats a lot, but only if he needs the fuel because he's worked or played hard.

He is a three-square-meal-a-day guy. He is fairly regimented in his eating. If he gets up at eight, he eats a hearty breakfast. Then he will eat at noon and again at six. There are very few times when he snacks, but if he does it will be one well-chosen snack, such as one Oreo. I don't think I've ever eaten just one Oreo in my life. He can and he does.

There is not a person alive who can make my husband eat something if he is not hungry. It doesn't matter if there is one piece of his favorite pecan pie left, he will pass it up even if I threaten to throw it away. He loves to eat, but food does not tempt him like it does me. A pan of brownies sitting on the kitchen counter does not call his name to come and consume its contents in the middle of the night. It never crosses his mind. If it is there, I can't get it off my mind. I will succumb to its call.

Bottom line: he eats normally. I eat abnormally.

The first year of marriage was both exhilarating and difficult for me. I had come from a great job with lots of close friends whom I missed terribly. I was sure a husband could equal 50 good Christian friends. Because I loved him and wanted to be with him, I thought once we were married I would have no wants or needs, ever again. I loved being with him, but I missed connection with friends who were 900 miles away.

> **Bottom line: he eats normally, I eat abnormally.**

Roy was working during the day and I wasn't, but not because I didn't want to. It was hard to find a job even though the town we moved to had several denominational headquarters and colleges. However, I wasn't a member of any of the denominations and the fact I had a degree from a different denominational college just called attention to that.

Money was tight. Even buying groceries was difficult. Roy said to me, "Whatever you do, don't skimp on buying groceries. We have to eat." I heeded his advice. Of course, he wasn't saying I should buy all the Twinkies and Ho-Hos in the town. But I translated it to buy anything I wanted. He was saying we have to eat three regular meals a day. We were speaking different languages and I didn't even know it.

At home with little to do, I ate. I did find a part-time job in the evenings at a radio station. I hadn't been there a month until Roy lost his job and we moved again to an even smaller town. Now I had the same problem all over again. I repeated the cycle, finding a part-time job at a newspaper. I was gaining weight. I knew it, but I couldn't seem to stop.

DISCIPLINED VERSUS UNDISCIPLINED

The honeymoon had started to wear off and it was time to buckle down and be an adult. When I was in Richmond, my life had been active. Then my excuse for not losing weight was I was too busy. In the first year of marriage, my excuse was I wasn't busy enough.

I had too much time with myself and filled it with worrying about finances, purposes and destinies. Sometimes it included whether Roy would get paid that week, and if not, where we would live the next week. He had four jobs the first year we were married and we moved three times. One would think that would have drawn me closer to God, but it didn't. I was spending no time in prayer and Bible study and lots of time worrying. Part of the worry was because I was spending money we didn't have and running up credit card bills to buy things like ... food.

I had too much time to myself and filled it with worrying.

I was undisciplined and lacked self-control. I wanted to eat whatever I wanted whenever I wanted. I didn't want anyone telling me what I could or couldn't eat. Not that anyone was.

It was just Roy and me. He expected me to be an adult and manage my own life.

Before we met, Roy had been in the Army, part of the time serving in Viet Nam. The Army taught him discipline. His father, a hard-working farmer, instilled a strong work ethic into his sons. By the time we got married, Roy was an adult in every aspect of the word. He knew how to manage his life and his appetites.

I hadn't had anyone in my life that consistently mirrored such attributes. My father demonstrated unconditional love, support and spiritual qualities. When I think about it, he was fairly disciplined in other areas, as well. I mainly connected to his spiritual qualities and his desire to spend his life working for God, whether it paid anything or not.

I looked to my mother for what a woman should be. Growing up she was so consumed with her emotional needs she was not able to model that. I never wanted to be weak like my mom. I never wanted to be angry. I never wanted to have uncontrolled emotions.

I equated my grandmother's way of demonstrating love with the wonderful food she cooked. Though a fabulous woman, her way of showing caring for me or any other person was cooking our favorite foods. How could I be disciplined when tempting food was placed in front of me? For me love was spelled f-o-o-d.

When a friend offered Roy a job closer to home in Jefferson City, we moved. I am sure I got the temporary job at the Missouri Baptist Convention (MBC) because of my work at the FMB.

My job was communications specialist. I worked directly with departments to write and develop brochures, posters, news releases and stories. The stories appeared in the weekly denominational newspaper.

I perceived a kind of competition mentality with many of the departments. Every department director wanted a front-page story in the paper. They wanted the best and biggest brochures to attract the most people to their events.

My job was salaried, which meant I got paid the same no matter how many hours I worked. I worked extremely long hours and many Saturdays. I did not feel appreciated for the extra work. As a matter of fact, I was asked to do more because they knew I would get it done. At that time the word "no" wasn't in my vocabulary. If my boss asked me to do something, I said, "Yes."

DIET CENTER®

During one evaluation, he told me if I wanted to do a good job in the office, it would be best if I wore nicer clothes and lost some weight. This concerned me. The job was a temporary position, which had been created just for me. He could decide at any time he didn't need a communications specialist. Losing weight would be good because my clothes were getting too small. Plus, I really did want to look nice for my husband.

I didn't want to give up my comfort foods forever, just long enough to lose the 100 pounds that I'd gained in two years since getting married. The pastor's wife at the church we attended had lost weight by going to Diet Center®. I decided to try it.

The plan involved eating exactly what God had been telling me whenever I asked Him what to do to lose weight. Namely eat more lean protein, cut out sugar, eat fruits and vegetables and limit starch. I found a few things I really liked on the diet and went with those. I ate a lot of skinned and deboned, baked chicken breasts, salads and squash cake made with eggs, squash and the center's special protein, along with lots of cinnamon and sweetener.

Primarily, it worked for me because they had a chewable protein pill to take between meals. The protein pill helped keep my blood sugar levels stable so I didn't have a desire to snack. I remember asking if I could purchase just the pills after I went off the diet, but they were only available if you were paying the weekly price for being on the program.

After about a year, I weighed one morning at home and saw the magic numbers pop up. I needed confirmation by the more sophisticated scale at the center. I went in at noon to see if the scale would show the magic 100-pound loss. When it did, I hugged the diet counselor and drove to work on cloud nine cranking the music as loud as it could go.

THE ELEVATOR

I got on the elevator with one of the departmental chairmen, a tall man probably in his 40s. At this point in time I was still in my 20s. I didn't know him well. I really never talked to him. His secretary was the go-between for any articles I needed to write.

He punched the floor number and then looked me up and down slowly. He said in a low, soft voice, "You look really good. I mean really good."

The air seemed to get thick. I was back on the trail to the creek. A Copperhead had just been spotted. He stared at me and continued talking. I couldn't speak. I froze. When the elevator opened, he looked me up and down again and said, "I'll be seeing you and I will be looking forward to it."

One could say I was hypersensitive and he surely did not mean anything unseemly in his remarks. Perhaps he was just trying to encourage me.

Whatever he meant, the remarks made me feel stripped bare. It was as if I had given up my suit of armor and was now vulnerable. The other nagging thought in the back of my ridiculous mind (that seemed to over think everything in detail) was if I hadn't lost weight, I wouldn't have tempted this supposedly godly man. It was my fault he lusted after me and, therefore, I needed to correct it by gaining back the weight. I proceeded to do this post-haste.

At break, I got a Butterfinger® candy bar out of the machine and a diet soda. I inhaled the candy in record time and went back for another. I didn't sit down and tell myself to begin to gain the weight back. It wasn't a conscious decision, but I can trace the beginning of gaining weight again to that elevator incident.

Fear took a firm grip on me. I was more scared of a man I saw only a few times a month than how gaining weight might affect my marriage. I was more afraid of him than of dying an early death. I was more afraid of him than of fulfilling the mission I felt God had on my life.

It's not surprising that in no time at all I gained the weight back, plus more. It was almost like my conscience had been seared in that area.[1] I didn't listen to any voices that told me I should lose weight. I ate whatever I wanted. I went through my daily activities, working, going to church, visiting with friends. We had weekly gatherings with other young adult couples. We bought a home. We got a cat.

We were dealing with everyday life of washing machine breakdowns, cleaning gutters and birthing kittens. I ignored my weaknesses regarding overeating and my fear of men who hissed.

I was frightfully out-of-control in the area of eating. I blamed it on protecting myself. I was a married woman. I loved my husband. We had a wonderful intimate life. I did not have to be afraid of other men, but I was. It was a childish fear.

On that elevator, I was an 11-year-old and a grown man was about to do things to me I didn't think I could stop. It was a flashback, but I couldn't ignore my feelings or reactions. It was a fear I should have taken to God. I hid behind a cushion of flesh. It was time to grow up, but I had no idea how to start.

THROUGH THICK AND THIN

My husband's desires that I lose weight and be healthy have always been born of love. He was always the opposite of the men of whom I was afraid. I knew he loved me, but I felt I still needed to protect myself against the other type of men. It was like obesity was my armor against the world of Copperheads that might appear at any moment.

Roy has a consistent, caring, easy-going personality. He is my solid source when the world seems to be turning upside down. He has loved me through thick and thin, more of the former than the latter.

The fact that we have been married forever attests to his commitment. This commitment has not been without trials and tests. What was about to come was one of those trials.

ENDNOTES

1. 1 Timothy 4:2, NIV

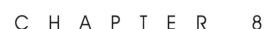

CHAPTER 8

TRASH DAY IS SO ROMANTIC

*"Love is patient and kind. Love is not jealous or boastful
or proud or rude. Love does not demand its own way.
Love is not irritable, and it keeps no record of when it
has been wronged. It is never glad about injustice but
rejoices whenever the truth wins out. Love never gives
up, never loses faith, is always hopeful, and endures
through every circumstance. Love will last forever."*

1 Corinthians 13:4-8 NLT

O ne day in the spring of 1983, about six years after my
wedding, I sat writing in my journal, a box of Girl
Scout Thin Mints in my lap. My husband was watching
television. He turned off the television and walked downstairs
to his ham radio lair. An hour or so later, I heard the back door
shut, the car start and back out of the driveway.

I knew he would be gone for the rest of the evening, most
likely to a fellow ham radio enthusiast's house. It didn't matter
what the weather was like or the time of day, if he wanted to
leave he would do it, not out of anger, but because he wasn't

used to reporting to anyone. It pointed out a great difference in us. He was quiet and independent. I was talkative and dependent. This was something we should have worked out a long time ago.

I began to ponder how that had happened. In the past we had deep, meaningful conversations over scriptures or our personal concerns. We went on motorcycle rides together and long drives. We talked about our dreams. Now we never seemed to talk or do things together. We had fallen into a rut, a ditch or perhaps a deep, bottomless cavern. It felt like we were two people living separate lives.

I had read articles about the first few years of marriage. I knew what I was feeling was common among newlyweds, especially those who had been single and living on their own before marriage. There was an assumption the mate would be Prince Charming or Cinderella or Mom or Dad. When they didn't measure up to the vision, things began to get stale in an everyday, bored sort-of way.

BLAMING WEIGHT

I blamed our seeming disconnection on my weight. I had gained what I had lost several years ago plus more. My weight was edging close to the 300-pound mark. Somehow I had rationalized anything under 300 was all right. Over that mark was bad. I wasn't at bad, yet, or was I? I hadn't weighed in forever. If I didn't weigh, then I could put the problem out of my mind.

It took some courage to step on the scale. The 330 shocked me. No wonder my husband didn't want to be around me.

Then it hit me. I weighed twice as much as my husband and I was nine inches shorter.

I wanted to fix things, and since the most obvious problem was my weight, I figured I would work on that and make a dramatic change overnight. (Insert magic cure alarm bells here.) Roy would see my effort and our relationship would magically be fine. In my profound wisdom, I decided to embark on a 1,000-calorie diet cutting out all sugars and eating only lean meats, vegetables, fruits and limited breads.

The next day I started a food journal. I ate 782 calories. Who knows how much I had been eating before. I had to be eating at least 3,000 calories a day just to maintain my weight. I was gaining weight, so I was eating that and more every day. My faulty thinking surmised if I could go back to the weight I was when my husband and I first met, we could recapture our honeymoon relationship. The trouble was, I was wrong.

My watchword would be: "If anyone, then, knows the good they ought to do and doesn't do it, it is sin for them."[1] I would keep it in mind at all times. I knew "the good" I should be doing. I looked down at the box of cookies. I knew I couldn't eat a box of cookies in one night and lose weight. I knew the right things to eat. I just didn't do it because I craved all the wrong things.

I had actually prayed for a Girl Scout to come to my door selling cookies. I don't know if God answered my prayer or not, but she showed up. I bought 10 boxes of thin mints and one of shortbread. The shortbread was for Roy. It would last him all year. Mine would be gone pretty soon. It was kind of like the children of Israel who complained to God because they wanted meat and bread. God was pretty mad about it, but He actually answered their prayer.

"They willfully put God to the test by demanding the food they craved … They ate the bread of angels; He sent them all the food they could eat."[2] They should have prayed for Girl Scout cookies. Then they wouldn't have gotten tired of manna.

I loved those cookies, but to be honest, I wasn't eating cookie after cookie because I was hungry. I was eating out of tension, worry and confusion with a lot of compulsion, boredom and habit mixed in. I knew what I needed to be doing. For some reason just the fact I shouldn't be eating cookies all night drove me to do it all the more.

THE EASY WAY

Don't get me wrong. I wanted to lose weight. I just wanted it to be easy. I wanted to eat the food I craved and lose weight at the same time. I didn't want to do the hard work. I figured I'd just get God to fix me. Relieve my desires to eat everything under the sun. Heal my weird emotional dependence on food and then everything would be perfect, especially my marriage. I was going to the right Source, but I was praying the wrong prayer.

I did want to do something to change the trajectory of my life. I lived to eat instead of just eating to live. When going to a friend's house for supper, the menu was the most important thing. I never missed a church carry-in dinner because there would be so much yummy food. I baked and cooked constantly far more than two people should eat. My husband ate a normal portion. I ate the rest. The food was never thrown out.

There was so much in me that was wrong. I felt like a garbage can. I had been dumping in the wrong foods, wrong thoughts, wrong desires. I prayed and told God it was time to clean my garbage can and make it look feminine. Really? I'm not sure how I expected Him to accomplish that.

Another issue was my emphasis on works, which actually drove my desire to eat. I was trying to do things so I could be a good Christian so I could have eternal life. This was wrong thinking. I had memorized Ephesians 2:8-9 and knew salvation was a free gift of God's grace and had nothing to do with what I did. Still it really seemed I had to do something to get God's attention. Although I knew the truth of the scriptures, I couldn't get it straight in my actions.

I was constantly asking God how to please Him. I even wrote a list about what I could do so God would be pleased with me. I am a list-maker. When I make a list, I check off every completed task. If all tasks are checked off, the project is complete. In my way of thinking, God would not be pleased with me if I did not do all 20 things on the list.

MY LIST

1. Spend time in Bible study, prayer and meditation every day.

2. Journal every day.

3. Stay on His eating plan.

4. Drink more water. Drink less diet soda.

5. Go to church. Go to Sunday School.

6. Practice and sing with choir.

7. Start a young women's group at my church.

8. Don't be prideful. Be humble.

9. Be a good wife, trusting, caring, giving, listening, understanding.

10. Be a good daughter. Go see Mom and Dad more.

11. Don't spend money unnecessarily.

12. Tithe. Give above a tithe.

13. Help the poor.

14. Be a diligent worker.

15. Love everyone at work.

16. Be a good witness and example.

17. Keep up with family and friends.

18. Share my talents by writing for religious publications, writing spiritual messages for secular markets.

19. Share my talents by painting pictures that declare God's beauty and goodness and wonder of His creation.

20. Be a good neighbor. Get to know the people who live around us.

Wow, what a list and it didn't even include the 40 hours a week I worked. No wonder I felt I could never please the Lord. I don't think anyone could ever do all those things at once. Yet, I felt I had to or I wasn't a good Christian. When I couldn't do it all, I felt guilty. Then I would eat.

I knew I should repent of overeating, but if I did it meant I was making a decision to turn from doing that because it would be in the category of sin. But eating wasn't a sin, was it? I mean everyone has to eat to live. I reasoned it away as not such a bad choice. I had a big list I couldn't complete. As a result, I had a lot of guilt. A lot of guilt required a lot of food.

After realizing I was failing at psyching myself up to lose weight, I joined Weight Watchers®. Once again, I was looking for the magic cure. I was not losing weight for myself. I was doing it to try to force something out of my marriage I felt was missing. Maybe if I lost weight, it would fix everything.

I added to my "doing" list, lose 30 pounds a month, exercise by swimming and walking, take the stairs at work and walk places. Once again, I added some pretty impossible tasks.

After a few months of effort, I gave up again. Nothing had changed substantially at home. I felt I was making this overwhelming sacrifice, but Roy saw little difference between 330 pounds and 310 pounds. Most people don't. I'm not sure what kind of change I was looking for in our relationship, but whatever it was it didn't happen.

FARTHER APART

I was trying harder, but we were getting farther apart. I felt I was giving and he was taking. He felt the reverse. Looking at the evidence, I have to agree with him. I was spending money right and left for larger clothes, more food, fast food, diet food and diet programs. I was saying I was trying to lose weight, but I was eating way too much food to be following any diet that would work. In my mind, I was giving my love to him by working hard and running the household. I thought he was a taker because it didn't seem he was interested in our relationship. His viewpoint was the more logical, but I had tunnel vision. I could only see my point of view.

We argued. We misunderstood each other often. We jumped on things the other said, which were not meant to be harmful or disrespectful. I, especially, wanted to solve every problem he brought up instead of listening to him or hearing his point of view. I would become defensive without really knowing why. Many times he didn't mean what I thought he meant. As a result, any type of communication seemed to end in hurt feelings.

Communication was a key we hadn't learned. We talked around, under and over each other, but not really listening, not encouraging or supporting each other. Because I became defensive, he stopped talking. We wanted things to work, we just had no idea how they could.

Eventually he talked about leaving. It never happened. We didn't have enough money for either of us to go anywhere. Even the fact we didn't have money was my fault. I spent a fortune on food and larger clothes, many times putting every day bills on credit cards. I was a failure and I knew it. To fix it meant I would have to give up eating junk, which was my way of coping with inadequacies. I had no idea how to rectify my issues.

I was a failure and I knew it.

Every time he would mention seeing someone we knew and how good they looked, I added the unspoken part of the sentence, "and you look horrible."

If he ever thought that, he didn't say it. I have an active imagination. I can make up my own conversation sometimes even swearing he said it out loud when I only surmised it from what he actually said.

My other way of coping was to try to reason with him. I told him how I'd stuck with him through job changes and bouncing paychecks. How I'd rejoiced with him through promotions and achievements. How I'd been there with him supporting every decision he'd made. I reminded him his best interests have been my best interests. I was trying to guilt him into staying. It only drove him further away. I knew we were losing touch; we literally walked around each other.

INTERESTING MEDICAL ADVICE

About this time, I went to a holistic doctor. I wanted medical advice about weight loss. I was hoping he'd fix my terribly mixed up body. I had been on birth control pills for years. He was against medications of any kind and suggested I stop and try a different form of birth control, which didn't require ingesting a pill. We took his advice and began using something called the birth control sponge.

That was in May. In early August I found out I was pregnant. I was large anyway and never felt sick or noticed much difference. I was astounded when I went for my regular checkup and the doctor told me I was pregnant and had been for at least two months. The next few months were perhaps the most difficult times of our marriage. If he hadn't felt trapped before, he certainly did then.

I wrestled with the possibility of being a single mom. I spent a lot of time alone or working. Our separate lives became even more separate. I read every book I could on marriage. I prayed more, studied the Word more and cried more in that season than ever before.

We had become part of a church, but weren't very well connected. I desperately needed fellowship and support so I went to a young women's Bible study. One night, I remember sharing that my husband and I were having difficulty in our marriage. I asked for prayer. I also remember the response. From that point on, I was treated like a leper.

During this time, most of my friends didn't want to discuss our problems. I felt they were taking Roy's side over mine. My sister, Renee, was my stronghold. I couldn't have made it through being pregnant and not knowing the future of my marriage without her constant love and support. She called me, listened to me cry and always told me it would get better.

MORE WRONG THAN WEIGHT

Roy was as stumped as I was about what to do about our difficulties. At times I thought if I could snap my fingers and lose 100 pounds all our problems would be over. Not true. There was more wrong than just my weight. I was a controller. I wanted to know where Roy was at all times. I would get angry if he didn't do exactly what I thought a husband should do. I stopped doing things I liked to do and started trying to do things he wanted to do. The fact I did these things only made me angrier when he didn't notice my efforts. We were for all intents and purposes, two single adults sharing an apartment.

We both believed marriage was a commitment for life, not to be confused with a life sentence. He agreed we should go to counseling as long as it was free and we had a male counselor. I agreed as long as the counselor was a Christian. I saw this as an indication he might want the marriage to work. I just wanted a counselor to fix our mess.

The first two counselors we saw were pastors who pointed fingers at Roy and told him he was wrong. He needed to love his wife as Christ loves the church.[3] Roy believed that, he just didn't know how to do it in the face of my obsession over food and my angry, manipulative and controlling nature. I wondered how I got off the hook with these pastors. After all, I was the elephant in the room and they were telling him he had to love me.

Finally we went to the free counseling program connected to the university where we both worked. The counselor helped us learn to communicate with each other. As I began to listen to what my husband was really saying, I saw the problem was not my weight gain, but my attitude. I had put Roy first in my life. I built him up, worshipped him, served him and mothered him. Who wants to be married to their mother?

When things would go wrong and he wouldn't be my king, I sought to fix him. My vision of a good marriage was the man who takes care of his wife, fills the car with gas, does everything on the honey-do list and then asks what else he can do. In other words, I wanted him to serve me hand and foot. When he didn't become what I wanted, I pushed harder by doing what I considered from my standpoint as love. I was really building a cage around him, from which he understandably wanted to escape at every turn. When he rebelled from my angry, controlling ways, I sought to enslave myself to other things: food, possessions, work, bylines, and positions in the church.

Roy's idea was an equal marriage where we both did our share based on our gifts and abilities. He actually tried to pull me up to learn new things, such as how to manage a budget and a checkbook, something I had never done well. He encouraged me to be my own person and not lean on him for everything. It was a more adult way of looking at things. I was looking for someone to take care of me, but do it my way. At one point in time, Roy told me in the midst of a discussion, "I am not your father and I never will be. I am your husband. There is a difference."

I finally began to grow up and start to become responsible for myself and rely only on God as my security, not Roy. If Roy decided to leave, I would be okay. I decided to put God first and although I wanted things to work with my husband, I let him go. I gave up. I realized it never was my job to hold our relationship together in the first place. It was God's.

SHOWING LOVE

During our counseling session, we talked about how couples get into a relationship and forget to do simple things for each other. The counselor gave us homework for the following week. We were to write down five quantitative things our spouse could do for us (other than any type of sexual relationship) that would show we cared about each other.

I remember only two things Roy wrote down. One was to turn off the hallway light before I came to bed. Another was to open the living room curtains during the day to let the sun in.

I remember two things I wrote down, as well. One was for Roy to mow the lawn or have the lawn mowed. The other was for him to take out the trash. He doesn't remember this exercise, but it was a defining moment for me.

The counselor gave us a tally sheet where we could mark down when our spouse did something on our list. I was diligent. Hey, it was a list. I can do lists.

The exercise gave me quantifiable evidence that Roy cared for and loved me. Every week since that day that he has been home on trash day, he takes out the trash. Every week he does, I smile. I love trash day. It's so romantic.

LOVE IS PATIENT

I felt a great relief. I was glad this meant my weight wasn't the major issue. I could learn how to have a better attitude, which I felt would be easier than trying to lose weight. I decided to focus on improving my love for Roy. I started with 1 Corinthians 13:4-8. It was a passage we had friends sing at our wedding.

I began reading the passage like this: "My love for Roy is patient and kind. My love for Roy is not jealous or boastful or proud or rude. My love for Roy does not demand its own way. My love for Roy is not irritable. My love for Roy keeps no record of when it has been wronged. My love for Roy is never glad about injustice, but rejoices whenever the truth wins out. My love for Roy never gives up. My love for Roy never loses faith. My love for Roy is always hopeful. My love for Roy endures through every circumstance. My love for Roy will last forever."

At every turn, I began to see how far short of the mark I fell. I would confess specific areas and ask God to show me more love for him. Tapping into the true Source can make any relationship last.

I was working on loving Roy, but I still wasn't admitting I had an addiction or life issue that gave me more satisfaction than my relationship with Roy or with God. I was not humbling myself before God. I was not washing my hands of any failures regarding food or even admitting I had done anything wrong. I knew I was overweight, but that's just the way God made me. I did love to eat. Losing weight and eating anything I wanted whenever I wanted were mutually exclusive. So I just shoved the desire to lose weight under the rug.

There were no tears or deep remorse and sorrow over my state. Well, let me rephrase that. There was sorrow over the fact my husband preferred me at a lower weight. He clearly saw I was letting myself be overtaken by a compulsion. He really didn't say it in so many words, but I felt he saw my weight as something I should be able to fix. I translated that as he cares more about our physical relationship than he does about me.

The predominant reason he wanted me to lose weight was for my health. He would be honest in saying he also preferred I look nicer, too. He never said these things unless I asked a pointed question and pushed until I got an answer.

What I read as his focus on my physical body at times made me feel he was reducing me to just a body and nothing else. It reminded me somewhat of the bad guys I had learned to stay away from. Deep in my heart, though, I knew Roy was one of the good guys. It just wasn't a reaction I could change easily.

TURNING POINT

Our son's birth was another turning point. He came six weeks early and had to be delivered by emergency c-section. It was necessary for him to be in the level two intensive care nursery. I couldn't leave the bed for 24 hours. The bed I was confined to would not fit in the small nursery.

Roy asked, "What can I do for you?"

"You can go be with our son," I said.

And so he did. He held him, sat by his incubator and reported his progress back to me. I was wheeled down to see him through the window. By the next day, I could go into the nursery via wheelchair.

Andrew had to stay in the Level 2 Neonatal Intensive Care nursery for 10 days. I was able to stay in the hospital for that time. Because Roy had the first 24 hours with his son on his own, the two bonded in a special way. The fear of being a good dad seemed to vanish when he held all five pounds and nine ounces of his own flesh and blood.

> I understood for the first time my weight was really not the core issue.

It would take several more months before Roy and I would work out our relationship. As he saw me become more independent and less clingy, he realized our marriage could work. I understood for the first time my weight was really not the core issue. The problem was multiple issues, including my insecurities about relationships, my suspicions, my jealousies, my pride, my fears and my bitterness.

WELL-MEANT WORDS

Buried down deep was my desire to lose weight. I just wanted it to be my choice rather than something forced on me. I knew my husband wasn't the only one who wanted me to lose weight. My grandmother was concerned as well.

Whenever I went to see her I could count on her to say, "Now, Honey, I wish you'd lose some weight. I'm afraid for your health. Here I baked you some oatmeal cookies, your favorites, I know." Okay, so maybe it wasn't run together in the same breath. There would be 30 minutes or so between the statements, but you get the picture.

Everyone wanted to run my life for me, but I was the only one with me 24 hours a day. Every choice was mine. Every bite I put in my mouth and every time I chose unhealthy food over what I knew to be a better choice was entirely my choice.

I could have said if my husband and grandmother wouldn't bug me about it, I'd lose weight, but I knew that wasn't true. I liked sweets and comfort foods too much. I needed them to keep me steady. I didn't want to live without them.

ENDNOTES

1. James 4:17, NIV
2. Psalm 78:18, 25, NIV
3. Ephesians 5:25, NIV

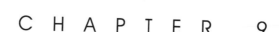

C H A P T E R   9

HUNGRY FOR IT ALL

"The angel of the LORD encamps around those who fear Him, and He delivers them. Taste and see that the LORD is good."

Psalm 34:7-8, NIV

"Why would anyone put an office on the third floor of a building without an elevator?" I asked that question to no one in particular as I climbed the stairs to my University Hospital office for the fifth time that day. It was a forced exercise program, along with walking to and from the parking lot on the other side of creation. At 380 pounds, I detested any unnecessary walking.

There were, however, advantages to having an office in the old building behind the hospital. As editor of the staff newsletter, I had peace and quiet to do my work, my own office and my own printer.

Another advantage was being able to have meetings there and receive visitors. Not many made their way back to my bird's nest in the trees, but when they did we could talk. One who stopped by from time to time was the advertising representative for the local Christian radio station. I was the public relations coordinator for our church and therefore had oversight of a small advertising budget. He would visit to see if we had any ads to place. We used the station's services quite a bit.

This day, though, he told me he had put his notice in at the station in order to start a Christian newspaper supported solely by commercial advertising revenue. I wanted to shout, "Wait! God gave me that vision. It's mine. You can't have it." Instead I smiled and mumbled my congratulations.

"The thing is," he said. "I need a lot of help. I need writers and editors because I need to spend my time selling ads. I really want it to be a quality publication."

I said, "You don't know this, but that's what I went to college to do. I have always felt this kind of publication is my calling. I will help you in any way I can."

He was holding a planning meeting at a friend's house. His friend was a photographer and writer who also wanted to help. We became the team that wrote, designed and published the newspaper. We helped him with two issues.

MY DREAM PAPER

His goal was to have a monthly free circulation newspaper delivered to supporting businesses and churches. He printed 10,000 papers, but could never deliver the bulk of them. Without a good distribution system, there was not enough advertising support to pay him a salary. He was becoming desperate for a job that paid the rent. In the meantime, a friend told me about a major Christian organization looking for a young man with a journalism degree, advertising experience and knowledge of African American culture. He applied, packed up and left for Washington, D.C. He bequeathed the Christian newspaper to us. All of a sudden, 14 years after God had shown me I would be editing and publishing a Christian newspaper, it was laid in my lap.

This was during a time of various Christian scandals with well-known televangelists. Each leader's fall was widely published on the front pages of our local newspaper. Our idea was to publish the good news, the many positive things that God was doing in the world, specifically in our area. The positive things never made it into our hometown daily newspaper. We would run articles about Christians making a difference, programs, churches, organizations and events.

We decided to increase the circulation and insert the paper, which we renamed *Good News Journal*, in our local newspaper. It would cost more to print additional copies and pay the insertion rate. However, it would be a built-in circulation so businesses would have a reason to advertise with us. We would also print enough copies to deliver to churches and businesses in our town and surrounding cities.

I became the main writer, editor and layout person. I decided the direction for each issue, assigned articles to the volunteer writers, edited stories and wrote many of the stories, especially the front-page articles. Being able to do this in the publication I felt I was uniquely designed to edit and publish was a dream come true. I also did the billing, oversaw the distribution and worked with volunteers.

My new friend mainly sold advertising and helped with some of the writing. She was also running another business from home, so life was busy for her, as well.

We decided to publish quarterly at first. We scraped by using borrowed computer equipment and printing things where we could until I purchased a Macintosh computer. That was in 1988.

As before, working for God began to take over my life. Finding what I loved to do, my sweet spot, made me want to work non-stop. Of course I still had a son, husband and full-time job. I was extremely active in our church discipleship program and teaching Sunday School. In addition, there was laundry, cooking, grocery shopping and house cleaning. Just like when I was first on my own in Virginia, I became overwhelmed with my life even though I loved it.

PROVERBS 31 WOMAN

I wanted to be the Proverbs 31 woman. I first heard about her at my great-grandmother's funeral when I was 14. The passage fit Mamaw, Grandma's mother, to a tee. When she was raising her children, she and her husband farmed. She kept everything in tip-top shape utilizing none of the modern conveniences we have today.

Whenever I think of Mamaw I see an image frozen on the big screen of my mind. She's sitting at her dining room table, her white hair bent over her big black Bible. Her face is reflected in the bureau mirror. Her back is to the door. It's her favorite spot to read the Word of God. The dining room table sports a white tablecloth with crocheted lace around the corners. The walnut-stained bureau has a short mirror and several flowers sitting over to the side. I inherited the bureau when I was nearly 40 and Mom and Grandma passed away within six months of each other. I had it refinished. It came out a beautiful burled oak.

That bureau sits in my kitchen today. It's the one piece of furniture I will have in my home as long as I live. It's the one thing I might try to strap on my back and carry out in case of a fire. That may sound rather obsessive. I suppose it is. I know Mamaw doesn't reside in the bureau; her soul isn't even there. However, when I look at the bureau, I'm reminded of her and the Proverbs 31 passage.

After the funeral, I went home and re-read Proverbs 31, a lot. I figured if this was who Mamaw was, I wanted to be that way, too. I wanted to be a Proverbs 31 woman.

Somewhere along the line, I even wrote my own modern-day paraphrase of the verses. I called it a paraphrase and personal goals. Really? Aren't goals supposed to be obtainable? I know if I lived nine life times I would never attain everything this particular woman did. I've heard, as you probably have, that this passage was a compilation of many godly women. Maybe that's true. I do know trying to aspire to be like her in all the traits she represents is impossible. I wrote the paraphrase putting my name in the woman's place and my husband and children's names in the various places. I got tired just putting the right names in the right places much less doing everything this super-woman was doing.

BURNING THE CANDLE AT BOTH ENDS

Though it was impossible, I tried to live up to all of these qualities. I was working at a full-time 40-hour a week job, which is 45 hours with lunch, and another hour a day to get to and from work. That makes 50 hours. Add an additional hour before and after work for delivering and picking up children. That totals 60 hours a week.

By 1990, *Good News Journal* was growing. We had increased circulation to 100,000 still not taking anything out of the advertising revenue for ourselves, but putting it back into the newspaper. With the increased circulation, we were distributing to a large portion of churches in about a 10-county area in mid-Missouri. Our volunteer distribution force had increased. However, a lot of the work still fell to me.

Still working for the newspaper, I was questioning how long I could continue. Our daughter, Jenny, had been born in June, and Andrew was about seven. There was now more work to do at home. That doesn't even count everything I was doing at church and writing what I could when I could.

> I was so enough God sent His son to die for me.

All of my trying resulted in some success, but mainly it just made me tired, frustrated and hungry, oh, so very hungry. The hungry part wasn't necessarily because I needed food. In all of this, I was looking for an outside validation that I was enough; that I mattered. I was trying to do something in order to be significant. It really didn't sink in that I already had God's validation. I mean I was enough. I was so enough God sent His Son to die for me. It was a free gift.

Yet there was this nagging feeling because of what He did, I needed to be more. I needed to do more. I hadn't attained the status of a Proverbs 31 woman because no matter how hard I worked I couldn't complete her list.

Growing up, I was expected to take on an adult role supervising my brother and sister, preparing meals, going grocery shopping, keeping up with laundry and doing house cleaning. I did this from about the age of eight, off and on until I was 18, depending on Mom's illness. I felt unprepared for the tasks at hand. It was a little like when I was six playing dress-up in Grandma's size 22 dress. I was swamped. I wanted to be big enough to fill that dress. If I were bigger, I knew I could do it all because Grandma did.

I had grown up. I was now bigger than a size 22. However, I still wasn't big enough to fill the shoes I had been given. How can you fill God-sized shoes? Can you imagine what size shoes He wears if the earth is His footstool?[1]

Although I never said these things out loud, and I didn't even think them consciously, they were part of my rational mind trying to figure everything out.

RIGHTEOUSNESS

In Proverbs 31, it does give an answer to the dilemma, yet I wasn't seeing it. "A woman who reverently and worshipfully fears the Lord is to be praised."[2] This type of fear is the beginning of wisdom and knowledge.[3] It's not fear at all, but a kind of reverence, love and respect for the Creator of the universe that should make me want to follow His ways. Of course, "there is no fear in love; but perfect love casts out fear, because fear involves torment. But he who fears has not been made perfect in love."[4]

I wanted to do everything the Bible told me to do, but I was missing the most important part. I was missing just reverently worshipping and loving God with my whole being—body, soul and spirit.

It's easy for me to worship God spiritually, especially when I am in church and the music is pounding a beat I love and words are deeply meaningful. It's even easy to do when I am driving along in my car listening to great Christian music or teaching. But where the rubber meets the road is to worship God by being the person He wants me to be; the one I was created to be.

From the womb, I was designed and knit together with everything I needed for existence.[5] This includes my body, soul and spirit. It's all there in an exceptionally unique package called me. I thought I had to be something more than who I was, though. I thought I had to be the super woman, leaping tall mounds of laundry with a single broom. When I couldn't, I beat myself up and tried working harder.

It didn't work. I was trying to fill the empty places inside of myself by doing more and more things. When I did, I ate more and more, which my subconscious did not think was wrong because I needed to be something more substantial. All along the Father was speaking gently to me. "Hunger and thirst after righteousness. Hunger and thirst after Me and you will be filled."[6]

David said it this way, "The angel of the Lord encamps around those who fear Him, and He delivers them. Taste and see that the Lord is good."[7] What did it mean to taste of the Lord? What would it mean to taste His sweetness instead of bread with sugar on it? What did it mean if I did that? How would I be filled? Would the empty places in my soul be filled? Would I be able to cease my endless cycle of work and more work?

FOOD THEY DIDN'T KNOW ABOUT

After Jesus talked with the Samaritan woman, the disciples came back with food and tried to get Him to eat because they knew He was tired and hungry. He confused them by saying He had food they didn't know about. They wondered who brought Him food. He told them, "My nourishment comes from doing the will of God, who sent Me, and from finishing His work."[8]

Jesus wasn't saying He was never going to eat. He had a physical body. He had to eat. He was saying what filled Him up was seeing His mission accomplished on earth. I felt I was accomplishing my mission on earth and yet, I wasn't full. I was always hungry physically.

How could I be as hungry for God as I was for candy? It didn't compute. And yet there was a yearning deep inside to do exactly that. I knew one thing; I couldn't be constantly working without taking time for recharging and refreshing. Working to the point of exhaustion slowed me down and made my family feel as though they were second place.

I knew I had God's grace, but what I didn't understand was how to employ His grace for power to do what I couldn't do on my own. How did it happen that His grace was like the engine? Where was the start button? I needed to find out because I was running on empty even though "fuel" was constantly going in.

ENDNOTES

1. Isaiah 66:1, NIV
2. Proverbs 31:30, AMP
3. Proverbs 1:7, 9:10, NIV
4. 1 John 4:18, NKJV
5. Psalm 139:13-16, NIV
6. Matthew 5:6, NIV
7. Psalm 34:7-8, NIV
8. John 4:33, NLT

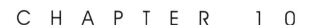

CHAPTER 10

IN SEARCH OF FREEDOM

"And you shall know the truth,
and the truth will set you free."

John 8:32, NKJV

I walked into the Freedom Seminar room to booming strains of *2001—A Space Odyssey*. The training assistants were dressed in suits and dresses, almost as if they were attending a funeral. I looked down at my standard black knit, elastic waist pants, oversize t-shirt and tennis shoes. Thankfully the others attending the seminar had on jeans and casual clothes.

If I hadn't known the seminar leader, if I hadn't been coerced into attending by some good friends, if those same friends hadn't paid my way, I wouldn't be giving up a weekend to bond with 23 people I didn't know. Personal growth seminar sounded so nebulous. But then my friends were so sure I should attend. The word "life-changing" was thrown around a lot.

I was told the seminar wasn't Christian, per se. I was leery. The cost was beyond what I could afford. I knew I had a problem with weight. I was a Christian, growing in my faith, even teaching adult Sunday School. On both the spiritual and physical front more "growth" was not what I needed. However, being set free definitely sounded good.

It was 1994. I had a 10-year old and a four-year old. I had quit my full-time job. I was doing freelance writing and still editing and publishing *Good News Journal*. The seminar would last for a weekend and then two weeks later continue for five days. I didn't see how I had the time to spare.

There was a pull towards going, though. I definitely needed something to help me climb out of the quagmire of flesh I had amassed. I had no idea if the seminar would help. I would go as a journalist, maybe do a story for *Good News Journal*. The seminar probably did deserve a story. Many were attending and finding it helpful. I decided I would observe, process and write about the experience.

The group members were varied, some younger and some older. They were in different stages of life—married, single and divorced. Their religious views were vastly different, Catholic, Protestant, atheists, Hindus, Muslims. Their sexual orientations were different. Their economic statuses varied. Some had careers, some didn't. Some were students, some had advanced degrees and some had never graduated high school. As a matter of fact, I would say I had never been thrown together with such a vastly different group of people before.

SHARING

During the first session of the seminar, I was convinced there was not one person similar to me. I was by far the largest one in the room. That wasn't such a shock to me. I almost always was the largest any place I went. Despite our differences,

I decided I'd give the group a chance, but I was determined just to observe. I wouldn't share. Many there had such earth-shattering problems. Mine seemed to pale in comparison.

I would get what I needed by osmosis. However, the seminar was structured in such a way that participation was inevitable. One of the first exercises was to pair with another person and share for two minutes on a specific topic. It was to be two minutes of talking without interruption. After that time, my partner could comment or ask questions. If I didn't want to talk or have anything to share, my partner and I were to sit and look at each other and wait for the time to be called.

Just when I got familiar with the routine of sharing, the trainer would shake things up a bit and have large group sharing or an active exercise of some type. Many of those attending had no qualms about sharing in the large group. That was still pretty far out of my comfort zone.

We ended the first weekend swaying to a song, standing in a circle with arms around people we had only met two days before. During the song, I looked around at the faces and decided if I ever did have something to share, I would tell this group. They could be trusted. I just wasn't sure what to share. I looked down at my body and wondered, what caused this? Would confessing my compulsive overeating do anything to help me lose weight?

In real life, I knew the trainer and his wife. Russ and Pat were ordinary people. Here in the personal growth seminar, they were stars with what seemed like supernatural insights. I was intrigued with their ability to somehow instinctively know what an individual was thinking. Actually, they only asked questions. The questions themselves seemed to reach into the depths of the person sharing, but each comment, each simple question, tugged at something deep inside me, as well.

FEEDBACK

During the second time-frame, things got deeper as we were led through exercises regarding each of our parents. We went to an imaginary pit. It could be any shape and design we decided it to be. We symbolically threw in things we felt were holding us back. I wanted to toss myself in, but then there would be nothing left. Separating my extreme morbid obesity from who I really was began to stand out to me as an almost irresolvable issue. If I got rid of the weight, who was I?

If I got rid of the weight, who was I?

One section of the seminar was feedback. Most people find this to be one of the best and worst experiences. After demonstration by the training assistants of what constitutes good and bad feedback, we got into our small groups of six to eight. As one member of the group stood, one at a time each additional member stood, made eye contact and gave them feedback.

It seemed mean to tell another person what I saw as a difficulty in their life. We'd been together for about four days, but we really didn't know each other very well. Of course, I had been observing and so I had some ideas. I thought I was ready for the exercise. I could take whatever was said to me. As a planner, I thought about what I could say to the others and before anyone else spoke, I was at the ready.

I remember each thing I said to others in the room. "You are using food as the only thing in your life you can control." (I think this person was anorexic.) "You are afraid of finding the beauty inside." (This person was wearing a lot of dark clothing.) "You are afraid of being yourself." (This person was extremely shy.) "You are being a victim." (An accident in which he was driving ended up taking his son's life.) "You are afraid of the real person." (He was hiding his sexual orientation.) "You are using anger to try to control your life." (She was angry about a divorce.)

Though I thought I was ready to receive feedback, I really wasn't. I figured they would say innocent little things that didn't really hit at what was going on in my life. I mean I was covering it up pretty good or so I thought. Everyone else in our group had cried; even the men shed tears. I determined I would not cry. It was my turn. I stood.

Then, the words came from each person. "You are hiding your beauty, intelligence and love inside by covering it up. You are pretending everything is okay when you know it is not. You are hiding behind a mask. You are using food as a control. You are using your eating disorder as an excuse for not revealing yourself to the world."

Okay, they didn't have to be like the facilitators and see through me completely. And where's the tissue box anyway? I didn't just cry, I blubbered. It wasn't because I thought they were mean; it was because they loved me enough to tell me the truth. The truth hurts, but fortunately it also has healing properties.

We wrote down what others told us and what we told others. Under what we told others, we were instructed to write: "This is my own personal feedback. I have to experience it before I can give it."

I knew everything I had spoken and others had spoken to me were on target for my life. It began to sink in my issue with food was more than just a love of certain types of food; it was in some way an emotional issue. It was a cry for help. It said, "I'm not all right and I don't know what to do about it."

I was playing the victim. I can't lose weight because I like food too much. I can't lose weight because Mom was crazy. I can't lose weight because an older man sexually abused me. I can't lose weight because I need fuel to empower me to work for Jesus. I can't lose weight because food has been the only thing that has always been there to comfort me.

I was hiding. I was covering up, but I didn't see there was any beauty inside. I only saw the scared little girl hiding in the attic away from her mom, the pre-teen running from the Copperhead man who threatened to poison her and the adult treading deep water to try to win the smile of God. It was easier to pretend these parts of me didn't exist. It was easier to eat candy. Candy helped anesthetize the pain; helped me forget any shortcomings.

Three key things happened to me during that seminar. I got over my fear of speaking in front of people. I bonded with people I would have shunned before the seminar. I glimpsed a vision of the person I was designed to be.

SELFISH

I was selfish when I worked long hours for no pay only trying to prove something to God. My selfishness extended to not going places with my family or when I did go with them, just staying in the car and reading instead of exploring with them. I surmised they wouldn't want me tagging along because I'd just slow them down. Really, I was lazy. I didn't want to exert the energy it took.

I was selfish by not spending time playing with my son or daughter. By this time, they had ceased to ask me to play with them because they knew I would be busy. What did I have to do that was more important than playing a video game with my son or dolls with my daughter? I could at least read them a book once in awhile, but I didn't even do that. I let my husband do it. He loved to read to the kids. What did I do with the kids? Oh yeah, I took them with me to deliver *Good News Journal* so they could carry the bundles inside the churches and businesses.

It seemed my supreme selfishness was towards my husband. I didn't do things with him. I didn't share his hobbies or interests. Sometimes I actually looked down on his hobbies as time-consuming and not productive. I didn't spend much fun time with him or my children because I just didn't know how.

I remembered something Roy had said to a friend. He said I should live at the office because I spent more time there than at home. It made me sad when I thought about it at the seminar. Why was I doing that? Did I really think God wanted me to ignore my family? I had two awesome kids who loved Jesus supremely and a husband who was a dedicated provider and father. What was my problem?

If I was at home my time was spent cooking, cleaning, doing laundry and caring for kids. At my present weight, if I wasn't working at home or the office, I had to sleep. I had no energy for much else. I only filled my time with something I thought was useful, like work or housework. I didn't play.

If I came home from work and my family was out playing somewhere, I would feel lonely because they weren't home. If they did something together and I wasn't a part of it, I would feel left out. But any loneliness I had was due to my own self-imposed isolation. During these times, it was just my bag of caramels and me.

I thought about how I could arrange my life better so I didn't spend such long hours at the office. Maybe I could even learn how to play.

A story Russ told during the seminar greatly impacted me. It's a story of a golden Buddha statue. It is based on a true story of a large golden Buddha statue located in Thailand but with Russ's personal touches. It went something like this.

THE GOLDEN BUDDHA[1]

A golden Buddha was located in a small village. The small village was known for miles around as the "Village of the Golden Buddha." The people were well respected because of the golden Buddha. They took their value and identity from living in the village of the golden Buddha. They were wealthy and prosperous.

All of the other surrounding villages also had Buddha statues but none was as fine as the golden Buddha. There was a time of peace and calm until bands of distant marauders began to destroy and pillage the various small communities. Afraid the golden Buddha would be destroyed, the villagers quickly decided to hide the statue.

They decided to cover it up. They got mud and mixed it with water to make a kind of plaster. They covered the Buddha, but not just with one coating of the plaster. Like anyone driven by fear, the villagers applied many layers.

There was no evidence of the gold. People were barely able to tell it was a Buddha. They felt it certainly was not a Buddha of any significance or importance. The hostile raiders simply passed by the statue, ignoring it, looking for real treasure.

The village was raided many times, but no one paid attention to the ugly Buddha in the center of the village. Years and generations passed. Those in the village of the mud Buddha had become very poor. They were laughed at because of their mud Buddha. They felt they had no value or worth.

Over the years the climate changed, the rains failed to arrive on schedule and soon people were dying. Desperate to find food and water, they decided to move south to a river valley so they could have water and raise food. They loaded all their belongings on carts to move to the new location. And just like most of us, they made sure to take their junk with them including the old dirty Buddha.

The going was slow because the road was treacherous. Nearing the location of the new village, the junk cart's wheel broke, spilling the contents. It was dark and the villagers decided there was nothing worthwhile in the cart anyway, so they left it and went on to set up camp.

All night one old man thought about the village's Buddha. He remembered stories he had heard his great-grandfather tell about a golden Buddha which used to sit in the center of town. He wondered could it be the same Buddha?

Early the next morning, the old man tried to get some of the villagers to go back and find the cart and the Buddha, but none would go with him. So he went alone. He trudged back to the place where the cart had fallen. He climbed down a deep ravine. There he found the old mud Buddha where it had struck a rock. The old man was sad to see the Buddha had been damaged. Just then the sun's rays reflected off a glint of gold where the mud plaster had cracked.

He excitedly ran to tell the villagers who came back to help him retrieve the statue. They lovingly carried it to their village. After the discovery of the gold inside the mud Buddha, the villagers removed the years of caked mud that had hidden the Buddha's shape and core.

The new village of the golden Buddha became prosperous and wealthy. They had found their true wealth.

APPLICATION

We heard the story while each of us was lying on the floor in a dark room. Quiet music was playing. We were asked to picture ourselves as the golden Buddha who had just been revealed to all the people in the village. How would we feel? My immediate answer was, vulnerable and exposed. I didn't have any idea of the real worth and value inside of me. I couldn't believe I was solid gold, worth millions. It was too impossible to wrap my brain around.

The story was one I couldn't get away from. It followed me for years to come. It is with me even now because the golden Buddha is me. I had good stuff inside, but I was hiding it under pounds and pounds of fat. What was I hiding? Why did I not want anyone to see or know the true me? Maybe I didn't even know the true me.

Coming to grips with the difficulties in my life helped me start to examine what I really wanted out of life. The inevitable time came during the seminar when I was challenged to decide.

"What do you want?" It was a simple question each person in the group had been asked. Now it was my turn. Just any answer wouldn't do.

Pat asked again, "What kind of woman do you want to be?" Earlier in the conference we had been given a definition of "holy." We learned the definition of the word boils down to "whole and healthy." In that moment, I realized that was what I wanted. I wanted to be whole and healthy. I wanted that definition of holy.

> I didn't have any idea of the real worth and value inside of me.

In discovering what I wanted, I also had to discover what I didn't want. Less than two years before that moment in my life, my mother had passed away. For some years, she had been a main part of our lives. She had gone through a process of healing and finally became the mother and a grandmother I loved and admired. Just when I was beginning to accept her position in the family and feel the wounds of my childhood healing, she died of colon cancer. One of her great attributes was the way she could remember every birthday, every anniversary, and every clothing size of everyone in our extended family, cousins, aunts and uncles. She didn't miss sending a card or a gift.

All family dinners and gatherings were held at her house. She had become the matriarch in every way. After her death, I felt the overwhelming burden of being that same thing to everyone in our family. I felt a little like when I was eight years old. Once again, I didn't know how to fill her shoes as the matriarch of the family.

I didn't know what I wanted, but I knew what I didn't want. I didn't want to be my mother again. I wanted to be me. I wanted to be free to love, but not in the same way she did. My group helped me feel free from that burden. Then I was able to accept my new contract with life. I was free to be a whole, healthy, happy woman.

Although in 1994 that seminar helped me define who I desired to be, it would take years for me to step closer to the full expression of what that means. On that day, in that seminar, I realized I had gold at my core. I had hidden it by years of muck and dirt, but it was there waiting to be found and set free from its prison.

ENDNOTES

1. Hardesty, Russell. "The Golden Buddha." Freedom Seminar. Columbia, MO., Missouri Board of Realtors Building, 2601 Bernadette Place. 12 November, 1994.

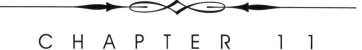

INSTANT PLEASURE

"Esau said to Jacob, 'I'm starved. Give me some of that red stew.' 'All right,' Jacob replied, 'but trade me your rights as the firstborn son.' 'Look, I'm dying of starvation,' said Esau. 'What good is my birthright to me now?'"

Genesis 25:30-32, NLT

I really had no say in the matter. The cardiac surgeon had told me in no uncertain terms I needed gastric bypass surgery. His nurse made the appointment. I had been called and reminded not once, but twice.

I figured I would show up and see what they had to say and be done with it. I didn't realize until the appointment this was a pre-surgery appointment, not an informational session.

I went in for a nice little meeting and before I knew it, I had been shoved into another one-size fits all hospital gown, poked, prodded, weighed, x-rayed and signed up for a surgery date. I was in a daze. The surgery date was less than a week away.

At the end of the visit, the doctor finally asked if I had any questions. I told him I was concerned about the small ring placed around the esophagus.

"What happens if I eat too big of a bite of food and it gets stuck?"

"The purpose is to encourage you to chew your food and swallow slowly."

"I get that, but what if I forget?"

"You don't want to do that."

"In a worst case scenario, what could happen?"

"You might have to have surgery to dislodge the food element. However, medications and other means would be tried first."

"In the meantime, I'm either gasping for air or hurting really badly."

"That could happen in a worse case scenario."

"I'm okay with every part of the surgery except the ring part. Can you do the surgery without that?"

"No, that's a part of the surgery. No alterations. One size fits all." He actually laughed at his joke. A little bariatric humor, I suppose.

DIETITIAN

The last leg of the visit was the dietitian. Bringing out a small saucer-sized plate, she displayed three plastic food portions. It resembled the kitchen set my cousins used to have. The portions were kid-sized as well: a meat patty about the size of a large silver dollar, a portion of mashed potatoes even smaller than that and a helping of plastic green beans that filled half of the plate.

"This is the portion sizes you will be eating," she said. "You need to start eating this way now to get used to how you will eat after surgery."

She continued talking about things to eat and not to eat, especially the first month after surgery. All I could think about was I could never eat just that baby portion of food. My daughter ate more than that when she was a toddler.

I knew if I could eat the way she was demonstrating, I would lose weight. I had tried the avenue of limiting myself and counting calories. It worked until I went off the diet and then began gaining weight again.

"Any questions?"

"What if I have this surgery and don't eat this way? What if I eat more food?"

"Don't worry. You won't be able to."

"What if I do?"

"Your body will react negatively."

"You mean I'll throw it up?"

"Yes, or it will get stuck. The ring on the esophagus won't let too large of an amount of food pass."

"What if surgery doesn't work for me and I still eat like I want to?"

"Why would you want to do that?"

The size six nurse did not understand my dilemma. It's not that I would want to, it was I knew I would if I could. I'd done it all my life. I hated being fat.

My purpose for living was entirely wrapped up in what I ate, how much I ate, where I ate and when I ate. Why I ate was inconsequential to me. In reality, I ate to protect myself, to make myself larger in my world and to bring myself back to an even keel whenever emotions got too far out of control one way or another. I had piled so much fat on my body, I didn't know who I was any more.

DEFEAT

I knew I could go to God for help in my time of need.[1] I knew He had blessed me with spiritual blessings.[2] I knew He longed to give me good gifts and wouldn't give me a rock when I asked for bread.[3] I knew when I was depressed I could go to Him and put my trust and hope in Him like the Psalmist.[4] I even knew He would help me when I was tempted to eat things, which were bad for me.[5]

I had graduated from a Christian college, studied the Bible, taught the Bible and took discipleship classes. The problem was not my knowledge. I had plenty of that. The problem was my vision. I had no concept or vision for my future. I could not see myself any other way than what I currently was, in the state I was currently in, being controlled by my desire for food, especially sweets and breads.

I related so much more to descriptions of defeat rather than victory. Romans 7 always seemed like gibberish to me. "I do not understand what I do. For what I want to do I do not do, but what I hate I do. And if I do what I do not want to do, I agree that the law is good. As it is, it is no longer I myself who do it, but it is sin living in me. I know that nothing good lives in me, that is, in my sinful nature. For I have the desire to do what is good, but I cannot carry it out. For what I do is not the good I want to do; no, the evil I do not want to do—this I keep on doing.

Now if I do what I do not want to do, it is no longer I who do it, but it is sin living in me that does it. So I find this law at work: When I want to do good, evil is right there with me. For in my inner being I delight in God's law; but I see another law at work in the members of my body, waging war against the law of my mind and making me a prisoner of the law of sin at work within my members. What a wretched man I am! Who will rescue me from this body of death?"[6]

ILLUSIVE VICTORY

I knew the next verse said victory happened through Jesus Christ. I even knew that Romans 8 gave me a recipe for living in the Spirit. It just seemed impossible. In this one area of my life, I was captive. No amount of tugging at the chains that bound me could set me free. It seemed to be a task too big even for God.

In college, I had memorized James 4. Back then, I rewrote James 4:1-4 to fit my circumstances. "Why do you want food all the time, even when you aren't hungry? It's because you have unfulfilled desires that battle within you. You want something but don't get it. You struggle and sneak what you think you want. You do not have what you really need, because you do not ask God. When you ask, you don't receive because you ask with wrong motives. You want to be set free instantly without pain or struggle. Then you can go on doing what you have always wanted to do, pleasing only yourself. You are cheating on your Lover God. Wanting to please only yourself means you do not want to please God. It actually means you hate

God. Anyone who chooses to be a friend of fleshly, worldly desires becomes an enemy of God."

As in all of Scripture, the answer is in the next verses. Their meaning and application seemed to elude me. It talks about how God opposes the proud, but gives grace to the humble.[7] On the outside I looked really humble. Actually I looked like a disaster waiting to happen. No one would suppose me to be proud.

Pride, though, seemed to be the only thing I had left. I prided myself on my accomplishments, on the Christian newspaper I published, on the articles I wrote, on the foster children I was helping, on my two awesome children and my loving husband. I was not proud of weighing 430 pounds. I was not proud of having a weakness I couldn't control, but desperately tried to hang on to what small amount of pride I had left.

Even the concept of submitting to God went over my head. I had already done that, hadn't I? I did that when I was seven and I also recommitted numerous times in my life. "Resist the devil and he will flee from you."[8] What if the devil seemed to be your own body that defeats you at every turn? What good is resisting an outside force if there is a stronger force inside?

> I was not proud of having a weakness I couldn't control.

There were two theological concepts I knew with my head but had no idea of how to apply them in the area of eating. First, the devil cannot indwell a Christian. Second, the Holy Spirit lives inside me and gives me strength and power.

The missing element in controlling my difficulty with food was my willingness to submit to God. I wanted to control it myself. I've always been a major control freak. I didn't trust others to be in charge so I stepped up and led. I didn't want to submit, so I tried to always be in charge. Then others had to submit to me.

God is the ultimate leader. For years, I prayed for God to intervene in my life and fix me. He was waiting for me to figure out I could only become healthy when I allowed Him to lead my actions and follow His teachings. Even when I did take action to lose weight, I did it so I could be in control. I would deny myself with diets for a season so I could lose weight and then go back to eating whatever I wanted. God was waiting for me to realize I needed His help. I still was not ready.

HIGH PROTEIN DIET

I did quick research and ruled out gastric bypass surgery. The next day, I called and canceled my surgery date. I was not ignoring what the cardiac surgeon said. I still wanted to live so I went back on the high protein, low carbohydrate diet. When I saw the doctor a month later, he was impressed I had lost 10 pounds. I let him know that I would be down 100 pounds within a year.

When I set my mind to something, I can accomplish great feats. I actually have a lot of willpower. Motivated by the desire to see my children grow up and live the awesome lives I knew they would live, I went back to eating meats and fruits. I didn't like vegetables and couldn't stand salads. I didn't cut out all bread or starches, but I greatly restricted them.

That was in the summer. By November, I had lost 60 pounds. My cardiac doctor was happy. I was still in the super morbid obese category. He encouraged me to continue the weight loss. My high blood pressure and diabetes were still being controlled by medication, but I was better.

I just needed to control my wants for a short period of time. Surely a person shouldn't be on a diet during Thanksgiving and Christmas. How could anyone celebrate those holidays without pecan pie, homemade fudge, sugar cookies, mashed potatoes, gravy and hot rolls with lots and lots of butter?

I went off the diet and began eating whatever I wanted. In the next two years my weight was all over the board. I tried many different diets and weight loss plans. One of the most intriguing was a plan that incorporated spiritual concepts with physical fullness. The basic premise was to eat when you are hungry and stop eating when you are full. I felt hungry all the time, but the plan said to feel true hunger. None of their concepts for what true hunger was connected with me.

Feeling full was another foreign concept to me. Though they teach that in the material, I could never feel where full was. I could eat supper and continue eating while I put away the leftovers. Within an hour I would be back in the kitchen for popcorn or to bake cookies. I wanted desperately to find full so I could stop eating. It never came and after not losing any weight, I stopped attending the class.

AMERICAN FAST FOOD

In the movie, "End of the Spear," Micayne, an Ecuadorian Indian, tells his wife about his visit to America. He says, "In America, they have little boxes with people in them. You drive up to the box and they give you food."

It is what I had come to expect from our instant society. It makes no sense to those in other countries. As an American,

I had bought into the concepts of immediate gratification and instant pleasure. I deserved to expend less energy to get what I wanted. I wanted to put forth no effort or energy and have everything done for me. I wanted to be catered to like a queen. Many times, I treated my children like servants having them go get snacks or sodas for me while I sat steps away on the couch in the living room.

There are pills to fix most any symptom an individual has. Surgeries cut out cancer and replace body parts. I wanted the thing that would fix me without much effort and I didn't want to give up anything to get it. I wanted to keep eating all the foods I craved and loved.

Immediate gratification is not strictly an American concept. Remember Esau in the Old Testament? He was so hungry he thought he would die. Jacob's stew smelled divine. He wanted some. Jacob said, "All right but trade me your rights as the firstborn son." This was a big deal back then. The firstborn got the blessing and the inheritance. He said, "I'm dying of starvation. What good is my birthright to me now?"[9] Esau's answer was one of instant pleasure not thinking about the future. He wanted something in the moment even if it cost him everything.

I had a foster daughter who had an extremely difficult time with this concept. If she wanted something, such as someone's dessert at work, she would take it. She risked getting suspended. Her mother said if she got suspended from work she would forfeit coming home the next holiday. I asked, "Do you love that dessert more than your mother?" She would answer, "No." I pointed out by stealing she was, in fact, choosing it over her mother.

The concept was beyond her because all she could see was the moment she was in. I was doing the same thing by choosing what I wanted to eat in the moment without thinking about the amount of weight gain it would cause in the long run.

My mother died at age 61 of colon cancer. I assumed I would be next in line. It was my lot in life. I was cursed. I was doomed. I was speaking into my own destiny with my thoughts. I was establishing my own destiny by my actions.

"Oh, wretched woman that I am, who can save me from this body of death?"[10]

ENDNOTES

1. Hebrews 4:16, NIV
2. Ephesians 1:3, NIV
3. Matthew 7:9-11, NIV
4. Psalm 42:5, NIV
5. Hebrews 4:15, NIV
6. Romans 7:15-24, NIV
7. James 4:6, NIV
8. James 4:7, NIV
9. Genesis 25:30-32, NLT
10. Romans 7:24, NIV, paraphrased

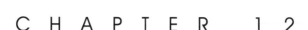

CHAPTER   1 2

LIFE OR DEATH

"And behold, an angel of the Lord suddenly
appeared and a light shone in the cell; and he
struck Peter's side and woke him up, saying, 'Get
up quickly.' And his chains fell off his hands."

Acts 12:7, NASB

The cardiac surgeon's words continued to ring in my ears. "Your heart was never designed to work in a body the size of yours." I was pretty stubborn, though. I didn't want weight loss surgery (WLS), but I was trying and failing at losing weight. I would lose, but then gain it back plus more, all the time panicking about what the surgeon had said.

I wasn't thinking about or praying about WLS. I had put that behind me. I was trying to ignore the possibility of such drastic intervention. It wasn't just not being able to eat things I wanted, the risks of surgery were extremely high. I had read about many different types of complications from nicked bowels to death during surgery. After the surgery, I would never again absorb all the necessary nutrients I needed from food. I would have to take various vitamins and minerals to get everything my body needed.

I would essentially be allowing surgeons to redesign my body. I would be saying, "God I'm smarter than You. I've got a better plan. So I'm going to go with this one." I accepted my fate and was busy living my life in the plus-sized world.

GARAGE SALE

School was starting in a month. I had two teenage foster daughters who needed plus-size jeans and t-shirts. Although they did have clothing allowances, they had used theirs for the year. The rest of the clothes needed to come from thrift stores or garage sales. I knew these type garage sales are few and far between so when I found one advertising plus-size jeans, I was excited.

We got there early, another necessity of finding the best picks. There were piles of jeans and tops in both of the girls' sizes. We found lots of clothes that might fit them. The woman let the girls go inside to try on some of the jeans.

I was intrigued about the amount of plus sizes the sale had. The woman there was about a size 10. I figured she must have a relative who was overweight.

I asked, "Whose clothes are these? I just wonder if they might have any more jeans in size 22."

"They're mine and everything I have is out here."

"Yours?"

"Yes, I've lost 100 pounds."

"How did you do it?"

"I had gastric bypass surgery last year."

"Really? I considered it, but I was worried about the ring they put around the esophagus."

"Me, too. They don't do that any more."

"Did you have any complications?"

"None."

"Did it really make you not be hungry?"

"Yes, it really works. There are times I want to eat, but I just can't."

"I was concerned about having the surgery, going through all the risks, re-routing everything in my system, not being able to absorb nutrients and then it not working for me. I'd be the one for whom it didn't work."

"That's funny. I thought that, too. It really can't not work. I mean you can jeopardize it by drinking shakes all day or something like that. It's just that with the smaller stomach, you get full really fast."

"That's my problem now. I'm never full."

"It was mine, as well. I'd eat a meal and then go back 10 minutes later and be famished. I'd eat all the leftovers and then start on whatever was available for snacking."

She told me about a seminar bariatric patients have to go to first before signing up for surgery. Her doctor required his patients to go to three seminars so they have all their questions answered before even thinking about surgery.

I figured it might be worth a shot. I put the card with the information on it in my wallet, paid $20 for well over $400 worth of jeans and t-shirts and went home. The plus-size garage sale was a Godsend in more ways than one.

Seed number one had been planted and began to find a place in the soil of my heart. Every once in awhile, though, I'd dig it up and carry it around and then decide to replant it. I wasn't fully committed to the idea.

RECOMMENDATION

Shortly after the cardiac surgeon's untactful declaration, I had talked with a friend who is a family nurse practitioner and told her my concerns. She agreed the surgery had some drawbacks and difficulties. She didn't like the ring around the esophagus, either. A few weeks after the garage sale she called me.

"I hesitated to call you because I didn't know how you would take what I'm going to say," she started the conversation. I encouraged her to continue.

"I was at a conference where they had a session on the new advances in gastric bypass surgery," she said. "The speaker talked about the exact problem you and I discussed with the esophageal ring. They have eliminated that from the surgery. The surgery is greatly improved and having excellent results. As a matter of fact, it is being considered the go-to cure for diabetes. I know what the surgeon said to you and I know your weight is back up close to or over what it was then. I'm very concerned about you. I think you should consider the surgery."

There was silence on the other end. I'm sure she thought I would react negatively. It took a lot of courage for her to call me. She didn't want to lose me as a friend. More than that, she didn't want me to die.

She sent me information from her notes and gave me the name of a local doctor who was doing the surgery. I thanked her and told her I would consider it. I still had one main concern. God made me a certain way with my stomach, esophagus and digestive system all designed to work. What does He think about gastric bypass surgery?

CHAINS

In the fall of 2003, about a month after my nurse friend called, my pastor, Gary Denbow, preached a very unique sermon. In the five years we'd been members, he'd never done an illustrated sermon. His sermons were always deep, theological, pointed and prophetic with words of knowledge sprinkled in. This sermon was going to be prophetic, but in a different way. God used that sermon preached in that way at that time just for me. Many others were also touched.

I don't remember the text of the sermon. The parts of it I do remember are very visual, which in itself is prophetic and a way God many times speaks to me.

Pastor Denbow held up a small gold chain and explained, "Some of the things which bind us are like this small chain. We can get over them ourselves. We don't need any help." And he snapped the chain. I thought of things like yelling at my children, which I'd made a conscious choice to stop.

He added that to break some chains we need other people to help us. He had a larger chain he tried to break and couldn't. He asked another man in the congregation to come and help him and together they broke the chain. It made me think of spending money on things I didn't need. I had gone to a financial planning seminar, which gave me knowledge and spiritual insight on how to do that. The trainers there were those who helped break that chain.

"Some chains need some additional intervention such as a treatment program of some type," he continued. He brought an even bigger log chain with a large cutter. While a man held it on either end, another man used the cutters to break the chain. Although I hadn't been to a treatment program, per se, I had been to Freedom Seminar. In many ways it helped me break some fears such as fear of speaking in public and of talking to those who were different from me. I wouldn't have been able to do that without the seminar.

"Still other chains," he said, "are so big they need a different kind of intervention." That's when he brought the largest log chain I've ever seen. It took four men to carry it to the platform! It was the type of chain used to tow a large truck. Two men carried a massive chain cutter onto the platform. It took both of them to hold it and attempt to cut the chain. They tried several times. The chain held fast and could not be cut.

He recounted the points. Some chains we can break ourselves. Some chains we need the help of our friends to cut. Some need the help of something like an intervention or treatment programs. However, there are those so massive, so entrenched, so binding, they can only be severed by a God-sized intervention. I immediately knew I needed a God-sized intervention.

That sermon was number three in the list of things I feel God used to get me to consider surgery. I needed to know it worked for someone. I needed to know a medical person I trusted agreed it was a good choice. More than all of those things, I needed to know God approved.

One of my big questions was, "Does God think it is okay for me to alter the body He gave me and made a certain way?" That Sunday God spoke to me in that still, small voice and said, "You have a bondage to food that needs a God-sized intervention."

During the prayer time I asked God if it was His will for me to have the surgery. I sensed while it was not His will for me to be super morbidly obese, it was His will for me to be whole, healthy and happy. I took that as a go-ahead to pursue the surgery.

> You have a bondage to food that needs a God-sized intervention.

RESEARCH

I began my research in earnest. I battled through the insurance process and finally found a hospital in my network willing to do my surgery even though it was 130 miles away. After being turned down by two of their surgeons, their head surgeon took my case.

I liked him immediately. He had a no-nonsense approach. When I asked about his mortality rate, he told me a couple of his patients had passed away after the surgery. However, he said they had pre-existing heart conditions. For them, the surgery was their last possibility for a life. He had been practicing for a long time and seemed comfortable with doing the surgery on extremely large patients. I agreed and a surgery date was set.

I had set my mind to have the surgery, but I was scared. The horror stories I heard made me cringe. I was doing this to live, not to die. One night prior to surgery, I read the memorials on a surgery website. These are tributes others have put online for those who either died having WLS or after. In most every case, the problems weren't due to surgical mishaps, but were because of issues such as heart and respiratory problems, which would have occurred whether or not the person had surgery. There also were some tragic stories of surgeons who bypassed too much of the colon requiring reversals of an already risky surgery. In some cases this resulted in a slow death. Leaks in the bowel and infection had also caused life-threatening difficulties.

I was at the end of my rope. I didn't want to live extremely obese. I was willing to risk death in order to live and be an active participant in life rather than a bystander. I also wanted to be able to do everything I was put here on earth to do. I was pretty sure that wasn't eating cinnamon rolls nonstop all day long.

I took the chance on having the surgery because I believed it was the only way I could be free of the chains, which had me bound. I wanted to really live, but at this point I was simply existing even though my life was full with family, church work, publications and ministry. I was miserable encased in a fatty living tomb. Like Peter, I longed to have an angel come and tell me to get up and the chains of obesity would just fall off of me.[1]

I was miserable encased in a fatty living tomb.

WLS looked like it just might be the magic wand that would make all my food issues go away. I would find out there is really no easy button to weight loss. By having surgery I was side-stepping facing the fact that certain foods had a stronghold on me. It appeared to me that the jungle of weight loss, food addiction and extreme obesity couldn't be navigated so I would have to have someone hack my way out.

ENDNOTES

1. Acts 12:7, NIV

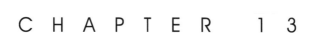

DENIAL AND MORBID OBESITY

"For, as I have often told you before and now tell you again even with tears, many live as enemies of the cross of Christ. Their destiny is destruction, their god is their stomach, and their glory is in their shame. Their mind is set on earthly things. But our citizenship is in heaven."

Philippians 3:18-20, NIV

I had RNY gastric bypass surgery in 2004. It was like most people said it would be. I simply couldn't eat large quantities of food even though I still craved everything imaginable. When I tried to eat anything more than say one-fourth of a chicken breast, I was so full I felt I would pop. It wasn't the full I felt before where I could stretch and unbutton my top button. It hurt. If I stuffed more in, it would come right back up because my stomach was too small.

If I ate anything with too much sugar it caused "dumping syndrome." For me, that meant I got extremely sick at my stomach, had cramps or diarrhea or both. That is not a good description though because it is unlike anything I've ever felt before.

Contrary to some opinions, during surgery a person's fat is not instantly removed to make a new improved model. Any type of WLS is a tool, plain and simple. I had been on every diet imaginable, lost weight, cheated and gained weight again. I had ordered weight loss supplements, took them for two weeks and stopped. I had bought an exercise bike, rode it faithfully for 30 minutes one day, then used it as a clothes rack until I sold it in a garage sale four years later for one-tenth of what I paid.

Gastric bypass surgery is a more invasive tool than any of these. It will last longer, but it can be circumvented just as easily. It took me about two years to lose 230 pounds, but that was a long way from the end of the story and the difficulties I would still face. It wouldn't be long until I had regained much of that.

EMOTIONAL EATING

Before surgery, I had always rejected the idea that I was an emotional eater. However, going cold turkey with all comfort foods had an immediate effect on me. It reminds me somewhat of second grade when my best and only friend in the world moved away. I cried for months. I missed being with her. I thought I could not live without her. I grieved her loss. It was the same with food. I missed my best friend—food.

Every place I looked I was reminded of the friend who had always been with me and I could always count on to help me through any difficulty. The sweet foods called to me from every grocery store aisle, every convenience store shelf, every fast food place on every corner, every carry-in dinner at church, every time we'd go out to eat, every birthday, wedding, graduation or holiday. I couldn't eat the things I wanted, but I still craved them and couldn't wait until the time I could eat them.

I didn't realize how much I relied on food to keep my emotions at even keel. I saw normal as a horizontal line. The objective of the game was to stay on the line. I didn't want to get angry and yell. That would be above the line. Excitable and joyous would also be above the line. Sad and depressed was below the line. Solemn and religious was also below the line. What was on the horizontal line was a kind of lack of feeling. It kept me living my life without emotional involvement because involvement was risky. I didn't want anything that didn't fit on the line. I didn't want to find out what might happen if my emotions got out of control. Food was my ticket to not having to find out.

If I could just have a good binge, everything would be fine. But no, I can't even do that.

There were times when I was angry. I didn't like myself then. It seemed others didn't like me that way either. I just wanted to be monotone, flat. Flat-line on a heart monitor means you are dead. I guess in a way I was trying to kill off any adverse feelings. Food, and specifically overeating or binge eating, is said to anesthetize pain. It helped me reach the flat-line. I didn't have to feel anything.

Feeling good made me feel guilty. Feeling bad made me feel pain. Neither was acceptable. With overeating removed from the equation, I had to learn how to cope with my feelings. I got mad at God because I couldn't eat. At times, I was like a raging drug addict who couldn't get a fix. Mostly I was silently mad and looking for ways to trick my body into accepting food.

I remember telling a friend, "If I could just have a good binge, everything would be fine. But no, I can't even do that."

WORK CHANGE

In 2005, we did a major shift from taking care of foster children to once again becoming a home for mentally challenged individuals through Department of Mental Health (DMH). This required a lot more work on my part.

Foster children require mothering. I knew how to do that. Record keeping is very minimal with Division of Children and Family. It was an entirely new ballgame with DMH. Paperwork, budgets, monthly reviews, daily logs and always more meetings seemed to grow by leaps and bounds.

By this time, I was publishing *FAMILY*, a parenting publication. We published 40,000 copies and delivered them to public and private elementary schools, churches and businesses in our town. The focus of the publication was parenting with a Christian slant. It was a free publication and so it was allowed in the schools. I started publishing this magazine when advertising sources dried up for *Good News Journal* in 2001.

I published *FAMILY* on my own which meant I had to sell advertising for it as well as write, assign stories, edit, design, layout, publish and distribute the issue. I also did billing for the ads. The paper was not a big success financially, but there were times when it made some money. I saw it as a ministry, not a job. DMH client-care was my business. All of it together was taking a toll on me again.

I was feeling better because I was losing weight. But I had not replaced my coping mechanism, which was overeating. Post-surgery instructions talk about finding new hobbies, something to replace eating. Chief among the suggestions was exercise.

I hated all exercise except water aerobics, which I had done on a limited basis. I really had no excuse not to go. I kept the gym membership current for my family and clients. So I started going sporadically. It didn't replace the comfort of food. I didn't think anything could ever do that.

I had tried eating some things with sugar, which made me sick during the first few months after WLS. Those experiences stayed with me long enough that I lost a large amount of weight.

DOWNHILL SLIDE

When I closed shop on *FAMILY* in 2008, I started reading a lot more. Many times it was research for something I was going to write. I like to eat when I read. It needs to be something easy to grab and shove in your mouth, like ... candy. Then it happened. I ate a Starburst®, one of my favorite candies. And then I ate another and another. Before I knew it the entire bag was gone and it hadn't even been a day. This started my climb back towards morbid obesity.

This is the weakness I knew I had, but I ignored its existence, kind of like an alcoholic who pretends one drink won't cause any harm. Eating that one piece of candy, took me right back down the path I had been on all my life, only now I had more at stake. I had greatly altered my digestive system to send anything I ate straight into the colon. Dumping syndrome had been a major problem but now it didn't seem to affect me. As I began to eat more and more sugar, my stomach stretched. These problems were less and less. I still couldn't eat a lot at one time but I could eat a lot by eating all day long.

I vowed I would not be one of the people who sabotage their WLS, and yet I did. I didn't go to the extent of where I had been but I was headed there fast. But by 2009, I weighed 260. I had gained 60 pounds. And I hadn't even gotten to the original goal weight I had set for myself.

DENIAL

Denial lives just across the street from morbid obesity. I chose not to look at my weight. I had knit pants that stretched with me. So what if I couldn't get into clothes I had worn only a year earlier? I've heard most everyone regains 20 percent of what they lose with WLS.

I didn't really hide the fact I was buying stock in Starburst®. I had also discovered cinnamon crunch bagels, which I bought by the baker's dozen because they were cheaper that way. I would put them in the freezer and microwave one whenever I wanted, which was often.

At five years after surgery, very few foods were off-limits to me. I still couldn't eat large quantities in one setting, but I could eat many times a day. That would have been fine if they consisted mainly of protein, vegetables and fruits, but my food choices held very few of those. I was sliding off the wagon, but I was acting like I wasn't.

There could be little denying something was going on with me, which needed to be changed. I didn't want to accept I needed to make major changes in my food choices. I rejected the idea I would have to give up some things for the rest of my life.

I was going to church, praying, reading my Bible and volunteering at local ministries. I was once again filling my plate to overflowing with both work and food. It was a dangerous combination for me. It would throw me back into deep waters if I did not get a handle on it.

MENOPAUSE

I was 51 when I had the surgery. Immediately I was thrown into full-blown menopause. I'm not sure if it was coincidence or a reaction to the surgery. Doctors, of course, say coincidence. Menopause wreaked havoc with me in every way. I was cranky, irritable, tired. I was experiencing mental fogginess and had no libido.

In addition, my main coping mechanism had just been severed. I could no longer eat my main comfort foods. That combined with the effects of menopause created a version of me I didn't like.

My regular physician prescribed numerous medications none of which worked. I read about compounded estrogen and testosterone sublinguals or shots. I found a local pharmacy that compounded supplements and asked what physician prescribed them.

They said the only physician in town prescribing them at the time was Dr. William Trumbower. A holistic and metabolic doctor, Dr. Trumbower is also an OB/GYN who delivered both of my children. The shot was what eventually worked for me. It put me back on track, restored my mental clarity and creativity, gave me more energy, made me more pleasant to be around and fueled my focus and determination. My shot is one thing I never miss.

I was now ready to tackle my weight issues in earnest. Coming out of the fog set me up to start on my journey toward victorious healthy living, which started in earnest in the following few months.

FLIP THE SWITCH

"All things are lawful for me, but not all things
are profitable. All things are lawful for me,
but I will not be mastered by anything."

1 Corinthians 6:12, NASB

"I don't know why it won't work," I complained to my son, the computer technician. "I followed the instructions."

"Is it plugged in?" he asked.

"Yes," I said, checking the plug again just to make sure.

"Is it turned on?"

"How do you turn it on?"

"Flip the switch."

"What switch? I don't see one. I don't think it has one."

"Look at the back."

I looked and sure enough it was there. And when I flipped it, the machine roared to life.

It's exactly like my journey regarding health. I didn't know where the switch was. I was plugged in spiritually. I prayed daily, read my Bible, attended church and taught adult Bible study. I was plugged in to my emotions. I desperately wanted to lose weight. I was going to die if I didn't. I was plugged in physically. I mean I was alive. I ate all the time, which was the main problem.

I had tried all the magic cures for weight loss, even the granddaddy of them all, gastric bypass surgery. I had no more tricks up my sleeve. I knew no abracadabra would fix my issue. Something else had to happen.

WEIGHT LOSS GROUP

When I heard a cognitive behavioral weight loss group was beginning, I attended the first meeting just to see what it was all about. The group was different from any other weight loss program, plan or diet of which I had been a part. It was designed to help us be accountable to whatever we set as our goals and to our plans to accomplish the goals.

No one told us what to eat, think or do. Through the meetings, various topics were presented. Then we discussed them as a group and talked about how the topic affected us specifically. At the end, we were encouraged to share what our goals were for the week. The next week, we'd share the progress on our goals and keep each other accountable.

There were no magic cures presented in this group, but there was magic to be discovered in the flip of my switch.

It happened for me the week the leader shared his story. More than 25 years before, he had been asked to lead a county program for DWI offenders. He was a counselor. He knew he could lead the program. The problem was he had an alcohol problem.

"I decided if I was going to lead this program and teach those who had DWI offenses about the advantages of being sober, I had to be sober myself," he said. "I would not teach something I did not practice in my own life."

He had been divorced twice. He didn't want alcoholism to ruin his third marriage. He had children. He wanted to start a positive legacy in his family. He wanted to be honest with those he counseled.

"I wanted my life to reflect what I teach and advocate," he said. "I knew drinking would negatively affect my life mission which is to call out the best in people." He made an agreement to do life alcohol-free with a sponsor and started down the road to recovery. He has been in recovery since.

CONNECTION

He mentioned something about alcohol being just one molecule away from sugar. This intrigued me. I had been thinking of the strong pull of sugar on my life, mainly candy, since I had started consuming it by the bagfuls again. Is there such a thing as being addicted to sugar? Is that even possible?

"What is the connection between alcohol and sugar?" I asked.

"Alcohol turns to sugar in the bloodstream. Many times when an alcoholic stops drinking, he or she gains weight. They go towards the sugar."

"So are you saying eating sugar is like mainlining alcohol?"

"Or vice versa. Alcohol is liquid sugar."

It hit me then. If an alcoholic can resolve his problem with alcohol by not drinking alcohol then I can resolve my problem with sugar by not eating sugar. My next thought was, "But I could never give up sugar." I didn't pursue it any more. The meeting went on.

At the close we were asked a simple question. What do you want? One woman said she wanted to lose 20 pounds. Her husband said he just wanted to support his wife. Another woman wanted to lose 75 pounds. Another wanted to learn to eat more mindfully.

WHAT'S YOUR PLAN?

When it was my turn, I said I wanted to be healthy for the rest of my life.

"What is your plan for becoming healthy?" I was asked.

"I will eat healthy and exercise." I knew as soon as that came out of my mouth it was a cop-out. There was very little measurable about that answer.

"How will you eat healthy?"

"I will eat more fruits and vegetables."

"What is one specific thing you will do this week towards that goal? And let me add, since you said you want to be healthy for the rest of your life, it needs to be something you will commit to do for the rest of your life."

The thing I knew I needed to say was I would stop eating sugar. I also knew it would be difficult. Sugar is in everything imaginable. So I went for my trigger food hoping I could make the next step later.

"I will stop eating candy." When I spoke those five words, the switch was flipped. It wasn't magic, really, and yet it was. I believe God was simply waiting for me to take the first step towards owning my addiction, my disease and my harmful life pattern.

Whatever words are used to describe the issue, one thing was sure, it had me bound in sweet, innocent-looking chains. For me, though, candy is anything but innocent.

During the session, the idea of stop-start had been discussed. That is, in changing harmful patterns, whatever I stop, I need to start something to replace it.

I was asked, "If eating candy is what you are going to stop, then what will you start?"

"Exercise."

"What kind of exercise?"

"Walking in the water." Good answer, I told myself.

"How often will you do this, when and for how long?"

I sighed audibly. Really, you want specifics? I've come a long way here. Give me some credit.

"When you have an appointment how do you make sure you remember to get there and don't schedule something else at the same time?"

"Oh, that's easy, I put it in the calendar on my phone which automatically goes to the cloud and connects to my home computer. So I have it everywhere. I really have no excuse for being late, um, like today." I laughed.

"What if you put exercise in as an appointment on your calendar?"

It was a simple, no-nonsense suggestion, but it worked. With my busy schedule of business appointments and meetings, client doctor appointments and my own appointments, my calendar was necessary. I had just been squeezing in exercise when I found time. It wasn't a priority.

SCHEDULING EXERCISE

By scheduling exercise first, I could build appointments around what benefitted me. I preferred to go to the pool during adult swim time, not because I don't like children, but because it's just easier to maneuver around adults. I scheduled exercise time every day for 30 minutes. I figured I could surely keep three of those.

The next week, I went to exercise five days. I loved the rhythm of walking in the water. I loved to meditate and pray as I walked laps around the water track. I soon built up to an hour, six days a week.

After three years, I am walking for an hour to hour and a half and stretching for 15 minutes. On days I have out-of-town meetings and find it impossible to get to the pool, I miss it terribly. I feel better, have more energy and get my instructions for what I need to get done for the rest of the day as I walk.

Walking in the water is also good non-weight bearing exercise. Since I still have issues with my knees and legs, it helps strengthen them and gives me exercise at the same time. It's an exercise that doesn't make me hurt while I do it.

When I can't get to the water, I ride an exercise bike or do an exercise DVD.

CANDY

The next week, I was at church. There is always a bowl of peppermint candies in the foyer. Peppermint candy is not a candy that tempts me. But out of habit, I absent-mindedly took one, unwrapped it and popped it in my mouth. Then I heard my own voice say, "I will stop eating candy." I spit it out and threw it away. I have had no candy since that time.

Several months ago, I was at the discount drug store and saw glucosamine chondroitin chews. I wanted to buy glucosamine to help with my joints anyway, so I figured I'd try this version instead of the tablets, which don't dissolve as well in my altered version of a stomach.

I took the box home, opened them and sat them on my desk. They did not taste like candy, but they were individually wrapped in gold foil. I found myself popping one in my mouth way too often. By the end of the day, what was a month's worth of glucosamine was gone.

I realized the chews reminded me of a habit of unwrapping candy and eating it. All of the candies I loved were the kind I unwrapped. Eating these didn't have so much to do with sugar as the process of unwrapping and eating candy. It was a neural pathway I had formed. To stop it, I just didn't buy them any more.

It's not that I think glucosamine chondroitin chews will take over my life, but each one has about 16 calories. There were 50 in the box. I consumed 800 extra calories in a day of something that didn't taste that great, but reminded my brain of something I crave. Sometimes I have to trick myself into doing the right thing.

STOPPING SUGAR

An amazing thing happened in the next few months. I stopped eating sugar. I did it on purpose, but I was surprised that it was not a difficult decision. Since I wasn't eating the concentrated sugar in the form of candy, it was not a painful choice to make.

This came about the same time as my birthday. My birthday is usually celebrated in conjunction with my niece and nephew who have birthdays near mine. It was easy not to eat cake and ice cream. I did eat a hamburger, salad and fruit. I found it easier to concentrate on talking to those present rather than worrying about whether or not I got the biggest piece of cake. In many ways, it was freeing.

On the way home, I rejoiced. "I did it. I survived a birthday without eating sugar. And the weird thing is, no one pushed desserts in my face. No one cared if I ate cake or not. It was totally my choice. And I was able to interact even more without eating so much."

At Halloween, I handed out fruit snacks. The holiday had always been more for me than for the kids anyway. I would choose my favorite candy. It was a chance for me to buy a lot of candy and then eat anything left over.

Instead I bought fruit snacks, which I knew I wouldn't eat. I felt better about giving semi-healthy snacks rather than concentrated sugar. I'm aware that some fruit snacks have lots of sugar. I checked the labels to get the least amount I could. The next week was a family dinner. I made sure the leftover fruit snacks went home with someone.

I had made the commitment to stop eating sugar, but at Christmas that year, I messed up. I didn't eat candy. No, this time it was sugar cookie dough. My daughter felt Christmas was not complete without sugar cookies. She made a couple of batches. The goal was to bake them and allow each family member to decorate their cookie. Everyone loved the idea and had fun decorating.

When I stay away from all sugar for long periods of time, I do not crave it. When I take one bite, I'm hooked again. I ate most of the leftover cookies. Fortunately, there weren't many, but it took several days before I came to my senses.

I realized I was not delivered from the pull of sugar. I may never be completely. When I get to the point that I think I am totally free, I find myself pulled in through the back door. For instance, a few months ago, I was at a conference. A friend was the caterer. She had dutifully put little placards on items that were gluten-free and vegan. By this time I was eating gluten-free, so I felt the peanut butter cookies she made were just for me. I knew they were not sugar-free, but I thought I needed to eat one in case no one else ate them.

> When I take one bite of sugar, I'm hooked again.

It was so delicious. I ate another and then another. When I went back to get some to take to my husband, there were none left. But there were oatmeal cookies left so I got several of those to take to him. On the way home, I ate two of his cookies as well before I heard that voice I have invited to remind me of my waywardness.

"Teresa, what are you doing?" It wasn't an audible voice, but I heard it just the same. I looked at the cookie in my hand, rolled down the window and threw it out. I processed why I had eaten cookies at that time when I had not done it in over a year.

BACK DOOR

One of the back doors for me is making sure I don't offend anyone. I think I get this from Grandma. It's one reason I will talk to complete strangers if I think they just might be someone I once knew. I'd rather talk to them than offend an old friend even if they aren't the person I think they are.

I felt the Holy Spirit whispering to me, "What's more important, your health or giving a friend a compliment by eating sugar, which really is something that can lead to your death?"

Now that I recognize this is an issue for me, I can deal with it. I am very up front about how I eat. No one can talk me into something I don't want to do.

There have been other relapses into eating sugar. But not overwhelming and never to the point I couldn't bring myself back to honor my agreement.

There is sugar in many things. I try to stay away from it. For instance, I love honey mustard sauce. The other day I happened to look at the ingredients in a packet and found no honey, only sugar. I looked in my refrigerator and sure enough the two bottles there were the same. They contained sugar, not honey. I find raw honey not addictive to me like refined sugar. I use it in a limited manner.

Sugar is processed. The processing alone can mess with my body. In concentrated amounts it is highly addictive to me. It is like a gateway drug leading to more and more and more until I find myself with hundreds of pounds of excess weight wondering how I got here.

ARTIFICIAL SWEETENERS

Diet sodas, Splenda® or artificial sweeteners also trigger my desire for sweets. They taste sweet, but there is no sugar high. My body wants the sugar high the sweetener reminds it of and goes looking for it. Thus, for me, artificial sweeteners are also gateway drugs.

An article in *Prevention* magazine agrees with me saying the more diet sodas a person drinks the greater their risk for becoming overweight. "Artificial sweeteners can disrupt the body's natural ability to regulate calorie intake based on the sweetness of foods. That means people who consume diet foods might be more likely to overeat, because your body is being tricked into thinking it's eating sugar, and you crave more."[1]

The chemicals in diet sodas are as bad or worse than sugar. Additional side effects are a two-fold increase in kidney decline specifically from the sweeteners, 34 percent higher risk of metabolic syndrome and cell damage from sodium benzoate or potassium benzoate and rotting teeth due to acid, according to *Prevention*.[2]

I was going through old letters recently and came across letters my husband and I had written to each other before we were married. I had sent him a note my friend had written called, "The care and feeding of a Tree," which, if you remember, was my nickname. One of her pieces of advice was to keep plenty of diet soda on hand. Gastric bypass patients are advised not to drink soda, but I started drinking it again when I started eating candy. I stopped drinking it along about the time I stopped eating sugar. I am living proof that diet sodas cause a person to gain weight by craving sweets.

Stevia is derived from a plant leaf so I do use it, preferably in its raw form. Lo-han Sweet® is another natural sweetener made from monk fruit. I also use this. Neither of these is addictive. My favorite way to sweeten anything, though, is through real fruit.

STOPPING BREAD

It was in the spring of 2011 when my switch was flipped in regard to cutting out sugar. The following August, I started hearing noises about wheat being bad for you. My two addictions have always been sugar and bread. If the two can be combined into such delicacies as cinnamon rolls or banana bread I loved it even more.

At the time I was going to a fitness trainer who was helping with some issues regarding my knee replacement surgery. I asked him what kind of eating plan they recommended. He said the paleo diet. This is essentially a gluten-free method of eating. The paleo advocate eats only meats, fruits and vegetables. All grains, sugar and high glycemic vegetables, such as potatoes and corn, are off limits.

I said, "I'm in the process of getting rid of sugar, but I could never give up my bread."

I should have known better than to make such a statement. I even mentioned the conversation to my weight loss group. The group discussed several people they knew who ate gluten-free and sugar-free because they saw it as a healthier lifestyle. Some were doing it for their children who had specific health issues related to gluten and flour.

It was basically another plant in my brain regarding foods that might be harmful for me. In essence I didn't have to ponder this long. I knew bread was something I craved and felt I couldn't do without. Therefore, I exalted it above God.

> I knew bread was something I craved. I exalted it above God.

The gradual approach had worked with sugar, so I cut out white flour. The decision always became firmer in my mind when I shared it with my weight loss group. I knew they'd hold me accountable and I'd either have to tell the truth or lie. I don't like to lie.

Cutting out white flour meant not making any more cookies, even made with sweetener. It meant no more hot rolls. I made the decision in September without really thinking about Thanksgiving or Christmas coming up. My house is usually the location for these events. Hot rolls were one of the staples I always provided at those meals. Nothing does my heart good like seeing something I've baked get eaten by the hungry crowd. This was the case with the fresh hot rolls.

I found wheat rolls, the same kind of rise and bake rolls I always got in the white flour version. I didn't find enough for the gang, so I supplemented with the white rolls. It worked and I stuck to my eating plan at Thanksgiving. I fixed a sugar-free pie with a nut crust. Others brought and ate traditional pies, but there were those who at least tried my sugar-free dessert.

People are watching for me to fail. Instead, they see me succeed.

I have to admit I did have a small sliver of pecan pie. It is difficult to resist when everyone is sitting around the table exclaiming over the great pecan pie a niece brought. The minute it touched my mouth, though, I knew it was too sweet for me. It nearly made me sick. It helped in a way to let me know my taste buds were slowly changing.

When I am honest with people and tell them I eat gluten-free and sugar-free, I have no issues. I have been doing this long enough I believe people are waiting to see if I go back on my agreement with myself. People are watching for me to fail. Instead, they see me succeed.

CRAVINGS

Early in November a friend and I were talking about inflammation in the body. I was still having aches and pains in my knees and legs. She told me allergies could cause inflammation. I had been thinking about that same topic, so I went to see her allergist, Dr. Laurie Fowler.

A month later I had the test that makes you feel like a pincushion. Afterwards I learned I was allergic to many things including bakers and brewer's yeast. Many times things a person eats or ingests will show up as stronger on the test especially if they are at all allergic. When I told the doctor I had never drunk alcohol, she was surprised because it showed up prominently on the test. She said it was even more of an indication I was extremely allergic.

Although Dr. Fowler recommends a healthy diet to her patients, with good variety, free of preservatives and processing, she said my test results showed it was imperative for me to stop eating anything with yeast.

In addition, she explained, foods we are allergic to present in one of two ways: things we crave or things we have aversions to. Foods people have aversions to are no problem because they don't eat them. The idea we are allergic to foods we crave got my attention, though, because I certainly craved sugar and bread.

I knew about acute reactions to things people are allergic to like peanuts, strawberries or even certain medications. An acute reaction can be anything from watery eyes to hives or an airway closing up.

I wasn't aware that chronic allergic reactions can affect any body system. Dr. Fowler explained allergies can cause many different reactions. This can be anything from not feeling well to inflammation in the body, joints hurting, nausea, behavior problems, cardiac issues, inability to lose weight, retention of fluid, extreme tiredness, skin problems, inability to think clearly and a myriad of other issues.

According to Dr. Fowler, those with extreme weight issues may have carbohydrate addiction and should stay away from sugar, as well as bread, pasta and other carbohydrates, which break down into sugar.

People crave what they are allergic to, she said. "If they stop eating the food they are allergic to, after a few months they won't crave it any more. If they do have some of it, they will find themselves craving it again. Craving is indicative of addiction. Anything someone is addicted to they are likely allergic to."

This explained why when I stopped eating sugar, I really didn't crave it. It also explained why when I stopped eating white bread back in September, I didn't crave it.

"Just try it for three months," she said. "See how you feel."

I decided to stop eating wheat altogether and go from there. I knew this was the right choice for me, but it would be difficult.

GLUTEN-FREE

The third confirmation came when I went to Dr. Trumbower for a checkup. He had mentioned eating gluten-free and sugar-free the year before. At the time I wasn't ready to hear what he had to say.

Now, though, I was all ears. He told me the benefits of eating this way and gave me suggestions about how to eat encouraging me to eat more beef since I was already taking iron supplements. He gave me a list of basic vitamins and minerals to take and suggested I get them from a health food store rather than a discount drug store.

He had the lab draw blood for a complete metabolic panel with several added tests he wanted to check. After getting the results, he added more minerals and suggested I start on natural thyroid pills.

Following my WLS, I had been able to stop taking my high blood pressure meds. Less than two years after the surgery, I had to go back on them. My regular physician told me I was genetically predisposed to high blood pressure and would always have to take them. Dr. Trumbower said chances were good I could go off the medications in about a year if I stayed on the gluten-free, sugar-free lifestyle and took the vitamins and minerals regularly.

It was right at a year later I was feeling dizzy. I took my blood pressure and it was extremely low. I called Dr. Trumbower and he weaned me off the medications. My blood pressure immediately registered in the normal range.

In three years, I have lost more than 88 pounds. I rejoiced the day my weight fell to the point I was just considered in the "overweight" category. It will take 23 more pounds before I am normal.

Although not everyone aspires to be overweight, it was a tremendous feeling when I hit that threshold. If I had not flipped the switch, I would be nearing where I was before I had gastric bypass 258 pounds ago. I shudder to think of the possibilities.

ENDNOTES

1. Oaklander, Many. (2012, August). 7 Side Effects of Drinking Diet Soda. *Prevention*. Magazine via Website.
2. Ibid.

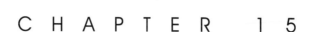

CHAPTER 15

BREAKING SWEET CHAINS

*"Beloved, I pray that you may prosper in all things
and be in health, just as your soul prospers."*

3 John 2, NKJV

W hen I made the decision to eat sugar-free and gluten-free, it was a decision for the rest of my life. Maybe I had just gotten tired of fighting my body and trying to make things work. Maybe I just gave in. Or maybe I knew the truth all along. I was a sugar addict, the same as an alcoholic only I didn't get falling down drunk and pass out.

My drug of choice was killing me, slowly but surely. The medical issues were closing in. I had prayed and cried out to God about this problem all of my life. I tried to fix it on my own. Finally I realized I can pray about this problem, but if I didn't do something different about what I ate, nothing different would ever happen and I would surely die.

Resistance or evil would win. I would be an easy opponent. He wouldn't have to work very hard to take me out of the game of life. All he would have to do is encourage me to do nothing except "gratify the cravings of my sinful nature and follow its desires and thoughts."[1]

One of the scriptures I have used as my watchword is: "Whether you turn to the right or to the left, your ears will hear a voice behind you saying, 'This is the way. Walk in it.'"[2] The verse says God will direct me when I'm moving forward.

The reality is if I do nothing, nothing will happen. Actually, if I do nothing, I go backwards. Remember the parable of the talents? The guy with one talent did nothing. When the master returned and heard he had buried the talent, it was taken away and given to the one who had multiplied his talents.[3]

I understand the guy who did nothing, especially if he didn't have a good plan. I want a plan. I want to know what the pieces are to any project and where they go before starting. I do the majority of thinking and planning on the front-end of a venture. Which means, I don't start many things.

My strength is in refining ideas, which is a good trait to have, but not so good if like the servant with one talent, I do nothing. When I continually refine and never start I become more entrenched in the mire of inactivity. What I had to do was stop figuring every single thing out and take a step of faith, not knowing what the result would be.

I couldn't wait until I figured it all out; I just needed to start in the direction of God's nudging. God had already been tapping me on the shoulder about some things I already knew.

FAMILY BACKGROUNDS

In a family of origin class back in the late 1990's I had mapped out both sides of my family, their birth and death dates and various information including tendencies and vocations.

My father's father and all of his brothers, my father's grandfather and all of his brothers, were alcoholics. My father's brothers were headed that way. My father was the one male in his family line that broke the curse of alcoholism. However, I knew the tendencies were still there in any descendants, including me.

On my mother's side everyone for generations back were hard-working farmers and robust farm wives with healthy appetites, obesity issues and type two diabetes. I remember my mother being very slim when I was a child. As she got older, she began to have weight issues and contracted diabetes.

I had known these facts most of my life, but seeing them on a chart was somehow disconcerting. I knew it represented a kind of compulsive nature on both sides of my family, perhaps even two different sides of some kind of weakness. There seemed to be a missing piece to the puzzle.

My father always warned against the evils of drinking. He felt it damaged his family. He wanted nothing to do with alcohol and drilled that into me. I made a conscious choice not to drink. Though some tell me it is crazy, I had a feeling if I ever discovered an alcoholic beverage I liked, I would be an alcoholic.

I always knew something was wrong with the way I ate. I was never full. I always wanted more. Following an eating plan without sugar and starches was impossible, but eating a diet with just a few of those things was also impossible.

When I realized I could be addicted to sugar and could live without sugar, I knew what my first step should be. Still, I was reluctant to place all my chips on that one assumption. What if I was wrong? What if it didn't work and I was a failure yet once again?

When I stopped sugar and most starches, I did it with a knowing in my gut and a quiet whisper from God that I was addicted. I didn't want to be addicted. However, the idea became very real when I examined how I felt about sugar. I craved it. I couldn't be without it. I wanted it constantly. I hadn't really researched all the ramifications, which is unusual for me. I just started in the direction and kept going knowing if it worked, I would continue it for the rest of my life.

SUGAR ADDICTION

When I began losing weight eating sugar-free and gluten-free, I decided to investigate literature related to sugar and alcohol addiction correlation. I was surprised to find there is a lot of information on the subject. Kathleen DesMaisons, an addiction nutrition Ph.D., talks about sugar and alcohol addiction in her book, *Potatoes, Not Prozac* and on her website, Radiant Recovery.

"You were born with a body that responds to sugar, alcohol and refined carbohydrates differently than other people," she says. "You are sugar sensitive. Sugar acts like a drug in your body. In fact, it affects the very same brain chemicals that morphine, heroin and amphetamines do."[4]

Knowing about your family history and tendencies is one thing that can point to the propensity for sugar or alcohol addiction. DesMasions says individuals may have this addictive personality if their mothers or fathers were alcoholics or had a craving for sweets. My parents both loved sweets, though they did not go overboard with them until later in their lives.

I still believe my family background points to the addictive metabolism because I have both alcohol and sugar issues on both sides to at least three generations.

METABOLICALLY BROKEN

The same body type that responds to alcohol differently also responds to sugar and refined carbohydrates differently. DesMaisons adds sugar addiction is "not a joke or a fad. It is a serious problem. If you have a sugar-sensitive body, you can be addicted to sugar. You can't not eat it. And because you are sugar sensitive, the 'high' you get from eating sugar is actually heightened."[5]

Sugar sensitive people are metabolically broken. They have unstable blood sugar, low serotonin and low beta endorphins, according to DesMaisons. With all three being out of balance the body reacts by wanting more sugar. It also contributes to such feelings as irritability, cravings, mood swings and sleep disturbances.[6]

> Sugar is not a joke or a fad. It is a serious problem.

Dr. Roberta Foss-Morgan in her article *Addiction to Sugar and Alcohol* explained it this way. "Sugar and alcohol addiction literally disables your ability to respond in a healthy way to your environment, cutting you off from the natural flow of good, which is called grace."[7]

I found Dr. Foss-Morgan's words to be more than true in my life. I knew what I should eat and how I should eat, but because I was addicted to sugar I couldn't seem to make it happen until

I admitted the addiction. Constantly feeling guilty about being overweight and having an issue with food put a block from accepting anything good in my life. I knew what a wretch I was. I didn't deserve anything good. God's grace was there all the time, but I was going to food instead of Him. The minute I admitted my failure and asked for forgiveness, I allowed His grace to flood my life.

ALCOHOL AND SUGAR

Tennie McCarty, founder and CEO of the eating disorder center "Shades of Hope," explained in the article, *Why Alcoholics Crave Sweets*, alcohol and sugar problems are so similar, which means their solutions are as well. "You can recover from sugar addiction, just like you can with alcohol and drugs, but first you have to be willing to admit and accept that it's a problem. The consequences from sugar addiction are different ... It's usually more the medical problems that will bring someone to their bottom."[8]

According to Foss-Morgan, alcohol is a liquid sugar. "Nearly 100% of those addicted to sugar/alcohol have abnormal five-hour glucose tolerance tests indicating this is a metabolic disorder. Some call this affluent malnutrition."[9]

She also says anyone born with this imbalance is "at risk of dependence on any drug that relieves the psychological, emotional and physical symptoms caused by being naturally medicated due to a deficiency in key neurotransmitters required for a healthy mind."[10]

Researchers have looked for the so-called alcoholic gene but they've come up empty-handed. The missing piece of the puzzle many believe is the metabolic disorder in how the body handles sugar.

It's difficult to ignore the evidence that sugar and breads cause addictive behaviors. It is a disease that overwhelms the body because of the heightened sensitivity to sugars.

Most articles say simply stopping eating sugar and refined carbohydrates is not enough. However, it is a step in the right direction. DesMaisons runs a center for alcohol and sugar recovery. Hers and other centers focus on a variety of avenues to help sugar sensitivity. My take away from their advice is to eat three square meals a day with lean protein and complex carbohydrates. Eat breakfast with good protein. Stop sugar. Stop grains. Move. Pray. Enjoy life and all its wonderful benefits. In essence, recovery includes becoming healthy—body and soul. I would add spirit, as well, for how can one come alive if they don't have the spiritual component?

SOUL NEEDS

"Beloved I pray in all things that you may prosper and be in good health even as your soul prospers."[11] This scripture leads me to believe the health of my body, even my broken metabolism, is directly related to the health of my soul.

The things my soul needs sometimes reflect negatively on my body, especially if I have not figured out what my soul needs. For instance, I may binge on sugar because I am feeling frustrated, depressed or happy and don't know another way to express it.

The fruit of the Spirit in many ways describes the things our soul needs that the Holy Spirit provides to our spirit as a fruit of His presence. These include: love, joy, peace, patience, goodness, faithfulness, kindness, gentleness and self-control.[12] I need all of these attributes in my life to feel complete.

Paying attention to what my soul needs keeps me from trying to find physical ways to meet those needs. If I am lonely, I may need to express love by spending time with people or calling a friend to talk. If my need is for significance, maybe I need to express kindness by finding a ministry, which needs my help. If I am upset, I may need to express gentleness by holding a baby or petting a cat or dog at the animal shelter.

I've found my exercise of choice to meet some of my soul needs. When I finish with my hour and a half in the water, I feel great. It is more than just a physical energizing. Exercise meets an emotional need I have of providing peace and soothing anxieties.

Beyond my exercise time, I need time alone to write. Interruptions frustrate me. Give me hours alone in a room just me and my computer and I am golden. Even the tap of the keys is like medicine to calm me.

Time with my small group also feeds a soul need for connection, communication, laughter and companionship. Oh yes, and we do study the Bible, as well.

Talking with or messaging both of my adult children gives me a thrill deep down inside. Of course, being able to actually see them and do things with them such as shopping with my daughter or hanging out with my son meets a soul need, as well.

I have a very soulful need to be connected to my husband, physically, emotionally, mentally and spiritually. There is something deeply bonding about a committed relationship.

Thankfully my five years of post-menopause apathy is well behind me. It is refreshing to feel that my husband meets my soul needs on many levels.

SPIRIT NEEDS

My high school and college years were during tie-dye t-shirts, bell-bottom jeans and the Jesus Movement. Contemporary Christian music was coming into vogue. My Christian friends in college told me I should break all my secular albums. I did that with every one of them, except Rod Stewart. (For some reason, he didn't count.) Anyway, I soon found I wasn't even listening to Rod, my favorite singer.

Christian music such as Love Song and Keith Green filled my ears because the songs filled my spirit. From that time on I have listened mainly to Christian music because I find it lifts my spirit and speaks to me like no other music can. I like all types of Christian music—contemporary, rock, rap, southern gospel, gospel, praise and worship, jazz and instrumental.

I also read, actually devour would be a better word, fiction and nonfiction Christian books to feed my spirit. I love to study the Bible, really dig into it and research it to understand more about it.

While strictly Christian movies are encouraging and feed my spirit, so does finding a spiritual application in a book or movie dubbed secular. In the car, I listen to podcasts or CDs from favorite speakers and pastors who challenge and encourage me. I love spiritual "aha" moments. I am active in my church, but feeding my spirit comes on a more personal level for me.

OTHER PHYSICAL NEEDS

To keep myself from feeling overwhelmed, I try to map out things I won't do. In other words, I intentionally neglect some things for a season in order to get a more pressing assignment completed. If I am working on a deadline, which is important to me, I realize I can't do everything. I have to pick and choose. I have to use the word "no" in order to maintain my health.

I have to use the word "no" in order to maintain my health.

I am beginning to recognize going without sleep to get something done does not help me. I am on this earth in a body. I have to "nourish and cherish my own flesh."[13] It's a given in the Scripture to do that. However, as a 21st Century American I tend to burn the candle at both ends. I have to get at least six hours of rest. I tried four hours and was useless the next day. If I get 10 hours I am tired and lethargic. Six to eight hours works fine for me.

I must eat three well-balanced meals a day. I cannot shirk on this or I will find myself in a desperate state again. Working long hours without getting good nutrition is part of the reason my body got in the mess it did. God does not want this for me. He wants me to prosper, succeed or thrive and be in good health. He wants my soul to prosper. If it is healthy, my body will be, too.

One observation about myself, and I think it is true of others who struggle with obesity, is I tend to put my needs last. This is wrong on many fronts. When I do this, I rob the universe of receiving the gifts God has placed inside me. Focusing on what

I need helps me help others. Spending some time thinking about my needs and wants is not selfish. It helps me be selfless. I can't shine when I'm not polished.

WEAKNESSES

It is true we all have weaknesses. Three times, Paul asked God to take what he called a thorn in his flesh away. And three times God said no. "But He said to me, 'My grace is sufficient for you for My power is made perfect in weakness.' Therefore I will boast all the more gladly about my weaknesses so that Christ's power may rest on me. That is why for Christ's sake, I delight in weaknesses, insults, in hardships, in persecutions, in difficulties. For when I am weak, then I am strong."[14]

I have often wondered if God doles out weaknesses in order to bring us closer to Him. My weakness for sugar and bread has certainly been a journey, which has made me more dependent on Him.

If Biblical fasting is a way to make me more dependent on God, then a fasted lifestyle should do that all the more. Giving up sugar and gluten-causing grains is a choice I made in order to be more healthy. It also draws me closer to God. I have to depend on Him to help me through each moment.

Something happened to activate the power of God's grace, and especially the fruit of the Spirit in the form of self-control, when I made the choice to give up candy. I made the choice to allow the Holy Spirit to be completely in control of my life. That means my spirit is now Spirit-led.

Not only that, I am in better touch with who I am and how God made me. It is a journey that will continue until the day I am called home.

ENDNOTES

1. Ephesians 2:3, NIV

2. Isaiah 30:21, NIV

3. Matthew 25:24-28, NIV

4. DesMaisons, Kathleen, Ph.D. "Are You a Sugar Junkie?" Radiant Recovery® - Dr. Kathleen DesMaisons, Author of *Potatoes Not Prozac, The Sugar Addict's Total Recovery Program, Your Last Diet*. N.p., n.d. Web. 24 June 2013.

5. Ibid.

6. DesMaisons, Kathleen. *Potatoes Not Prozac*, New York: Simon & Schulter; 2008. Print.

7. Foss-Morgan, Roberta. "Addiction To Sugar And Alcohol." Addiction to Sugar and Alcohol. N.p., n.d. Web. 24 June 2013.

8. McGuiness, Kristen. "Why Alcoholics Crave Sweets." The Fix n.d.: n. pag. Print.

9. Foss-Morgan, Roberta. "Addiction To Sugar And Alcohol." Addiction to Sugar and Alcohol. N.p., n.d. Web. 24 June 2013.

10. Ibid.

11. 3 John 2, NKJV

12. Galataians 5:22-23, NIV

13. Ephesians 5:29, NKJV

14. 2 Corinthians 12:9-10, NIV

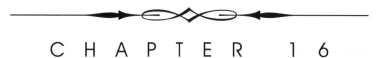

EASY BUTTON

*"No trial has overtaken you that is not faced by others.
And God is faithful: He will not let you be tried beyond
what you are able to bear, but with the trial will also
provide a way out so that you may be able to endure it."*

1 Corinthians 10:13, NET

I walked into the grocery store knowing exactly what I needed: eggs, chicken, rice, broccoli and strawberries. Inside the door, the first thing I saw was the pastry display. Donuts were predominantly displayed behind glass self-serve doors. Before I knew it, I had a plastic bag in one hand, the tongs in the other, my cinnamon buns picked out and put in the bag.

I had just made the decision to eat gluten-free and sugar-free. I hadn't been tested much regarding my decision. This day, the interior chatter in my brain sounded something like this, "You are tired. You are hungry. You deserve a cinnamon bun and while you're here, get two, maybe even three. You need them. You can always start that eating plan thing again tomorrow. Just this once won't hurt."

I recognized my own voice talking me into something I had decided I would not do. It wasn't necessarily the voice of the enemy. It was my own voice born of years of giving in to an area of weakness. I could only blame myself.

Don't get me wrong, I've always believed in the devil and his legion of demons that are out to tempt me with the eventual goal of stealing, killing and destroying.[1] He is the master of resistance, but most of the time his closest ally is me.

Many times I am my own worst enemy. Any time I attempt to start something beneficial to my health, I meet resistance. There are forces arrayed against me in the pursuit of any great challenge. Some of these include: fear, self-doubt, procrastination, addiction, distraction, timidity, ego and self-love, self-loathing and perfectionism. Another is rational thought.[2] Steven Pressfield talks about these in *Do the Work*.

Resistance occurs when I try to undertake "any act that rejects immediate gratification in favor of long-term growth, health or integrity. Or, expressed another way, any act that derives from our higher nature instead of our lower,"[3] he says. No wonder I have always had a hard time losing weight. The resistance is too strong.

This resistance comes from within me. I've blamed so many things for my weight gain. I blamed the awesome cooks in my family. I blamed poor knees so that I couldn't exercise. I blamed just wanting to eat all the time. I blamed everything, but myself. However, there really was no one to blame, but me. It was my fault.

That means I am the only one who can do something about it. So I start and then I meet resistance. I am not overwhelmed, though, because it is just a sign that what I'm trying to accomplish is vitally important. Now my goal becomes to overcome resistance. This is done not by sheer force of will, but with God's help and a plan of action including doing something everyday towards the project's completion.

WHY BE HEALTHY?

At Freedom Seminar in 1994 I declared that being healthy was a major goal in my life. Even after that declaration I still didn't live like it was. So in reality, it wasn't.

The key for me was to focus on how being healthy would allow me to move closer to the number one goal or passion in my life. When I did that, all of a sudden becoming healthy moved from just a good idea to something vital in my life. It became the most important thing in my life for several years and still is of prime importance.

For a time I went to a trainer every day, a physical therapist twice a week and a chiropractor once a week on top of exercising six days a week for at least an hour. I saw doctors and specialists as needed. I determined to make my health a priority because if I didn't, I wouldn't be here to do anything else. Health became my guiding star.

My number one passion has always been to write stories that matter. Because I couldn't really make as much money as I wanted doing that, I began to take care of foster adults. I did this for three reasons: to be home for my children, to have time to write and to make money. Of course, it helped that I didn't have to worry about walking long distances from a parking lot to work. I didn't have to be concerned about taking a nap in the middle of the day if I wanted to. I could eat anything and everything because it was accessible.

Please do not misunderstand me; I love the young ladies who live in our home. I'm good at doing everything it takes to operate a home for them. However, along the way in the midst of taking care of everything and everybody, I lost sight of my main passion and stopped writing.

When I looked at my life, I was far away from what I was designed by the Creator to do. This saddened and depressed me, but I didn't know what to do about it.

PASSION REVIVED

During a course on leadership, one of the assignments was to write a personal vision and choose a project to complete based on that vision. The powerful part of this exercise was realizing I thought my vision had died.

When advertising revenue dried up for *Good News Journal* and then *FAMILY*, I experienced a profound amount of grief over the loss of what I felt was my life purpose. I resigned myself to the possibility the vision had run its course.

I had told my group that my vision was helping others learn to write, but that was only part of it. It also included writing stories about real people living real lives going through real struggles connecting with a real God. I would publish these on a website.

I knew this was connected to my life verse, Habakkuk 2:2-3. "Write the vision. Make it plain so that those who read it may run with it. The vision is for an appointed time ... It will not tarry."

The era of the newspaper was coming to a close. Online was where writing was blossoming. The stories would have a reach that could only have been dreamed of in the print media. I knew this was something I could be passionately involved in. I continued taking care of foster adults, but I also worked at getting a new website up and running and beginning to write stories about people.

AIR BOOKS

As I began developing the website, I pushed another part of my purpose to the back of my mind. In 1998, I had seen a vision. Because of the place I was when I saw the vision, I thought it was specifically for one church and one time. When it didn't come true there, I tried to forget it. I couldn't because it stayed in the back of my mind where it resides even today.

In the vision it was a sunny day. I was walking through a field with tiny yellow and white flowers dotted throughout when I came upon a split-rail fence. As I began to climb over the fence, I looked up and saw three large books in the air just above my head against the backdrop of a beautiful blue sky.

The first book was a red book with very ordinary binding. It looked like an average library book. It was on the left side. On the right side was a gold book. It was the same size as the red book. In the middle was a very large silver book. This book pulsated with life. Glitter, sparks, actions, even conversations were falling from it.

The dream relates to three categories of books with which I will be involved. The red book tells of historical events related to redemptive activity. The gold book contains the truths of God made plain so they can be understood. The silver book's meaning seems to be about living life God's way with power and purpose. This is why it is alive.

A strong desire of mine has always been to write books. The actual doing of it seemed too difficult. I can write a newspaper article or a blog post, but an entire book? It appeared to be impossible. It also seemed presumptuous for me to say I had a vision to do this when I really had only written one book. It was an easy book to write because it was simply paragraphs of marriage tips for women. I wrote at the request of a friend who distributed it, along with one of his, back in the 1990's.

I realized if the full aspect of my life's vision was ever to be fulfilled, I had to start action towards it. My passion of writing books was renewed and activated. I knew I had to have my brain firing on all cylinders. I needed energy to carry out my task. I not only needed to be healthy, I wanted it in the worst way and would do anything to get it. It became more important for me to do my God-given assignment of writing than to eat a cookie or a piece of homemade bread.

I keep this vision in mind. Keeping the vision in front of me helps me resist temptation.

PUT THE BREAD ASIDE

Several holidays ago, I decided I should eat a piece of homemade bread a friend had brought for the meal. No one had even cut the loaf yet. I didn't want her to feel bad. It would be rude for no one to eat what she worked so hard to make. She might feel slighted. I cut the loaf and ate a piece and then another, resulting in almost 400 calories I did not need.

It's not that I don't ever make mistakes and veer off my eating course. Instead of berating myself for mistakes, I try to learn from them. I learned from that incident and others that homemade bread is a big temptation, especially hot, homemade bread and rolls.

There is a buffet my family and friends like to frequent. When the waitress brings the two baskets of huge, buttery, hot rolls and sits them down in front of me, I instantly move them to opposite ends of the table. I set the bread aside so it won't stare me in the face.

> Instead of berating myself for mistakes, I try to learn from them.

There are habits I have formed through years of eating what is bad for me. In visiting, laughing and talking I could without thinking grab a roll and start eating. Instead, I put temptation out of my reach.

Being a sugar and bread addict became an easier thing to manage once I realized not all food is necessary for survival or for the furthering of a friendship. If a friendship cannot survive me not eating a piece of homemade bread then I probably need to dig for a deeper root problem in the friendship.

KNOWING LIMITS

The other day, a friend suggested we meet for lunch at Panera's. I explained I couldn't go there because Panera's, for me, is like going into a bar would be for an alcoholic. She thanked me for telling her that and was fine with meeting elsewhere. After all, the reason for meeting was not to eat. It was to catch up on each other's lives. That is a true friend.

I know my limits. Why knowingly tempt myself? If I do go somewhere I am tempted, I try to think through the menu items to choose one that both satisfies me and keeps me within the boundaries I have set for myself. When I do that, I feel much better physically, emotionally and spiritually.

When I was a kid, I wanted the power to choose whatever I wanted to eat. When I became an adult and did just that, the food I chose turned on me and overpowered me. The very thing I thought I had power over actually had power over me.

It would happen the same for other addictions such as alcohol, drugs, tobacco, pornography, gambling, shopping, work, television or a myriad of other things. These are addictions I could choose, just like food, to anesthetize pain or escape emotional discomfort. If I did, one day I would find what I chose would have power over me. Suddenly, I would be out of control. I would be weaker than the thing I originally chose.

Many people feel as if they have super powers and can handle these things in their lives. Some can. However, when participating in any behavior becomes something I cannot control, it is an addiction. If I think I can't live without the substance or behavior, I am addicted. When I can't cope with everyday life without it, I am addicted.

The good news is, God knew this about me all along. He didn't leave me without resources. He gave me all the power in the universe. The same power that raised Christ from the dead lives in me.[4]

Many times I looked at my body and felt even God didn't have the power to help me with my problem. I felt disgusted with myself and hated what I had become. Was my body bigger than God?

All along, though, He was bigger and had the power I needed. All it took was faith on my part to trust His answer and then action to take the first step towards living a fasted lifestyle.

Although it sounds like a simple answer, I can tell you from experience, it is anything but easy. A friend of mine says, "If it was easy, we'd all do it. When are you going to do the hard stuff?"

For years, I was waiting for the easy button to float down out of the sky and fix me. I tried all types of things I hoped would allow me to continue to eat anything I wanted and lose weight at the same time. The truth of the matter is, this solution does not exist.

> If it were easy, we'd all do it. When are you going to do the hard stuff?

All types of weight loss programs told me they had the answer. Some worked better than others, but in the final analysis, they all take hard work. The only way I can hope to do the hard work is to set my face like flint[5] towards the goal of being healthy and pray continually during the midst of temptation.

STRESS RELIEVER

Recently, I had one of those extremely stressful weeks trying to get a lot of things done for my job. Since I run my own business and had some people on vacation, I had to manage extra shifts. I was ready to give in to some kind of eating binge. I had long since cleaned out my refrigerator, freezer and pantry of any offending items. I was seriously contemplating a trip to the grocery store to pick up a yummy mix of anything sweet when I heard the still, small voice, the One I had invited to remind me when I was tempted. He said, "You need Me. You do not need sugar. You are not physically hungry."

I found my Bible and looked up the verse that was rolling around in my head. "No trial has overtaken you that is not faced by others. And God is faithful: He will not let you be tried beyond what you are able to bear, but with the trial will also provide a way out so that you may be able to endure it."[6]

I put on some worship music and spent a few minutes journaling my thoughts, the reasons why I was contemplating an eating binge and some alternatives to the binge. I could go for a walk. I could write some more. I could read a Christian book. I could call a friend. I could watch a movie with my husband. I could go shopping for shoes I needed. I could study my small group lesson. I could go for a drive to nowhere specific.

Because I had been inside most of the day, I felt God leading me to go shopping. When I followed through with that action, it got checked off my to-do list, which helped clear one thing out of the overwhelmed column. It also released some restless energy. I came back home the long way, driving through the countryside. This always helps clear and order my mind.

Many times when I am tempted to eat something off my chosen lifestyle plan and solve the problem with a binge food, it is because a basic need of my soul or body has not been met.

As I pay attention to my needs, I am not tempted to eat off my chosen lifestyle plan.

Six months ago was the last time I ate off my plan. Before that it had been about six months. Each time I process through what I did and why and make a plan to not do it again. It's not, "I'll never do that again." It is, "Here's what I will do to handle that next time this or a similar situation happens."

Giving in to temptation is happening less and less frequently for me. I get stronger in my resolve as I meet each situation not with an attitude of defeat, but with one of victory. I say, "Okay, that's one more temptation I can check off the list because I know what led me to succumb to it and how I will handle it next time." My brain is being rewired with new neural pathways as I overcome temptation every day.

MEETING MY NEEDS

God made me a triune being. I have a spirit that wants to be connected to God's Spirit. I have a body. It is physical and requires rest, nutrition and activity. I have to meet those needs or it will rebel. My wanting to binge was not because I needed food. It had to do with a soul need, an emotional and mental need.

I was feeling overwhelmed, frustrated, stressed and knee-deep in work. These are the times I am most likely to turn to food. Instead, I followed through with taking a mini-vacation. I needed to change the scenery, to take a deep breath and feel a moment of peace. I needed calm. I needed order in the face of what felt like chaos.

When I go to Him for help in my time of temptation, He promises to give me a way out, but I have to do something as well. I have to listen to what He says and then follow through. Sometimes it's as simple as stopping and asking myself what I need.

Once I listen and follow-through with what the Holy Spirit speaks in my heart and what I read in the Word, it empowers me to withstand the next temptation. With His help I can do it again and again and again.

If God is for me, who can be against me?"[7] I am strong when I can clearly see His vision for my life and know I am headed there with His help. With His power I can be bold. I can say, "Move over temptation. Be quiet resistance. I'm coming through."

ENDNOTES

1. John 10:10, NIV
2. Presfield, Steven. (2011). Do the Work: Overcome resistance and get out of your way. Do You Zoom Inc.
3. Ibid.
4. Romans 8:11, NIRV
5. Isaiah 50:7, NIV
6. 1 Corinthians 10:13, NET
7. Romans 8:31b, NIV

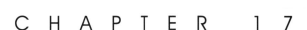

CHAPTER 17

POWER FOR THE POWERLESS

"The Spirit of the One who raised Jesus from the dead is living in you. So the God who raised Christ from the dead will also give life to your bodies, which are going to die. He will do this by the power of His Spirit, who lives in you."

Romans 8:11, NIRV

Recapping my weight loss journey should not be difficult. For some reason, though, I refused to look at all the facts. My highest weight was 430 pounds. I had gastric bypass in 2004 and by 2006 had lost 230 pounds. I weighed 200 pounds. By 2009 I had gained back up to 260. Once again, categorizing me as morbidly obese.

In the meantime, my weight loss group went through the famous 12 Steps of Alcoholics Anonymous and applied them to food. This is not a new concept. Overeaters Anonymous has done this for years. I was somewhere in the midst of losing about 10 pounds of this latest weight gain when step one came on my radar. I admitted I was a sugar addict and began my journey towards health.

STEP ONE

I value my independent nature, my ability to control things, my power over my choices. I did not want to take step one. It says, "I admit, I am powerless over food and that my life has become unmanageable." Anyone who knew me when I was at my highest weight knows this was true.

At our weight loss group, the leader was asking questions about how much weight I'd lost and regained and what I wanted to lose. I hedged adding 20 or 30 pounds here or there in what I had lost and gained to make it look better on my behalf. I couldn't remember from week-to-week what answers I had given because they seemed to change as often as I changed clothes.

> I needed to own my dilemma, but I was in a fog of denial.

I needed to own my dilemma, but I was in a fog of denial. Remember, denial is the next-door neighbor to morbid obesity.

To say I was powerless over food was an understatement. To say food had become unmanageable in my life was truer than true. Even at that juncture, I fell under the spell of any cake I baked, any cookies I made, any candy I bought, any supper I fixed. Even after gastric bypass surgery, comfort foods managed me; I certainly had no power over them.

The recognition of defeat was overwhelming. I resisted it for several weeks. The rest of the group was actually on step three before I could go back and fully admit my life had become unmanageable. Reluctantly I agreed with step one. I did not want to admit I was powerless, but it is true, I am powerless without God. I knew it in my head, but I finally fully owned it in the core of my being.

STEP TWO

I had tried everything known to man to conquer the thing that so easily ensnared me again and again and again.[1] I needed Someone to help restore me to sanity.

Insanity is something I know about. Although my mother did rally and make something out of her life during her last 20 years, insane is a term that could easily have been used to describe her. It was the family secret we didn't talk about. Some knew, of course, but we just didn't want to say, "She is crazy." It was not socially acceptable.

I had become like her in many ways. I had created my own kind of insanity. It said it in black and white right there in the 12 steps. Step number two: I come to believe that a Power greater than myself can restore me to sanity.

The truth is everyone needs a power greater than them to intervene and meet them at the point of their needs. When I was seven years old, my desire for candy eventually led me to accept Jesus' gift of eternal life. I had no idea 50 years later that I still would not have discovered the incredible power of that gift. Did I believe the same power that resurrected Jesus from the dead could help me stop eating sugar and stop gaining weight? Yes, I believed He could help me, but I knew I was the one who would have to stop putting the food in my mouth.

STEP THREE

Step three says I made a decision to turn my will over to the care of God, as I understand Him. To me it means more to say it like this. "I made a conscious adult decision to turn my stubborn will and my desire for sweets, candy, cinnamon rolls, breads, gravies, mashed potatoes, pasta, cheesy dishes over to the care of God as I understand Him." I was about to understand a great deal more about Him than I ever did before.

I relied on food to get me through any crisis, to be a comfort, to be a friend, to love me, to reward me, to accept me and even welcome me as a morbidly obese person, to always be there in any circumstance.

When I had WLS, I understood this tendency in part. However, I knew others had said even though one couldn't eat as much after the surgery, the process could still be sabotaged. Part of me said this tool will help me obtain my goal and force me to do what I need to do. Another part said I can still eat what I want, just less of it. Of course, I ended up listening to that last part.

It was a big risk allowing God to be my everything. I had always held something back in reserve in case God didn't come through. I always had food to turn to. To take step three meant it was just God and me.

My past failures at losing weight and keeping it off led me to know if I go back to inactivity or less mindful eating, it will lead to a disastrous outcome. I know how to sidetrack the weight loss process and get it off course.

I'm good at that, but not proud of it. I've admitted to God, my family, my friends, my weight loss group and now to you,

I have an area of weakness I am powerless over. I need help being restored to anywhere near sane.

I have turned my life completely over to the care of God, my God, the One who has been there all of my life, the One I've ignored, the One who didn't beat me over the head because of my failures but gently, lovingly, patiently worked to lead me to the place where I could surrender everything and start over.

Something dynamic happened when I surrendered, agreed with God that I had a big problem and repented of it. This time, repentance was real. This time it involved action. I turned around and began walking in the opposite direction of eating everything I wanted whenever I wanted. I began exercising even when I didn't want to. I repented. God saw it and said, "This is good."

> I gave up the food I thought I couldn't live without.

I gave up the food I thought I couldn't live without. I actually grieved thinking of never eating sugar or bread again. Feeling I could not live without it was the first clue I was addicted, allergic, bound and chained.

GRIEVING

Going through the steps of grieving included denial, anger, bargaining, doubt, acceptance and hope.

First, I denied this could really be my problem. Then, I got angry thinking about never eating these things again. I bargained with God saying things like, "Can't I eat it just this once?" Each time I'd do that, I'd see very clearly how addicted I was. Bargaining took care of the doubt.

I accepted my issue. I implemented a plan that worked for me. Seeing the plan work led me not only to hope I would be successful, but also to actually begin to see the realization of my dream.

THE DREAM

Many people told me in order to lose weight I needed to visualize myself thin and trim. I tried, really I did. Although many times I see pictures in my mind, that picture would not come. I couldn't for the life of me imagine myself thin.

I could, however, see myself in my wedding dress. One day I would fit into the dress again. It seemed impossible, but it was the only tangible thing I had. I could look back at wedding pictures and see the reality that I really had fit in that dress.

A dream backed by an action plan fueled by accomplishment takes on a life of its own.

Recently I did just that. I put on the dress. And it fit and was perhaps even a little loose.

As Napoleon Hill said, "Our only limitations are those we set up in our minds."[2] I accomplished the dream because a dream backed by an action plan fueled by accomplishment takes on a life of its own. When I begin to see it, nothing could deter me from the course set towards the fulfillment of the dream God had already seen fulfilled.

"God can do anything, you know—far more than you could ever imagine or guess or request in your wildest dreams! He does it not by pushing us around but by working within us, His Spirit deeply and gently within us."[3]

My thinking is too limited. I couldn't believe He would help me finally fit into a dress I'd already worn once. What more does He have in store for me? I can't begin to imagine, but I'm excited to find out.

<u>ENDNOTES</u>

1. Hebrews 12:1, NKJV
2. Hill, Napoleon. *Think And Grow Rich*. Los Angeles: Renaissance, 2001. Print.
3. Ephesians 3:20, MSG

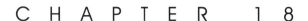

CHAPTER 18

GRACE, IT'S NOT JUST A GIRL'S NAME

"He gives more grace to stand against such evil desires. That is why Scripture says, 'God opposes the proud, but shows favor to the humble.'"

James 4:6, NIV

O ne morning in 1994, just before I woke up, I had a dream. I saw the Father in the heavenly realm sitting on a throne in a sort of palatial room. Jesus was sitting at His right hand. All around was a presence that was alive with what I could only describe as the sound a cold, blowing winter wind makes as it howls outside. I could see that God the Father and Jesus were shaking their heads and conferring.

Down way below them was the earth and extremely far away was me in my house. I was easy to make out because I was gigantic to the point I was afraid I would tip the earth off its axis. I was stuffing food into my mouth while I madly worked at my computer trying to get *Good News Journal* done. I had already moved the deadline back once. I couldn't do it again.

My immediate interpretation of the dream was that God was angry with me. Number one, He was angry because I was eating and overeating was a sin. Number two, I had not finished the paper on time.

It was a painful dream because I wanted to please God. I thought from the atmosphere of the dream that God the Father, God the Son and God the Holy Spirit were really angry with me. I had managed to raise the ire of all three persons of the Trinity. Who does that when they are trying hard to work in ministry and do what God wants them to do? Apparently, I did.

My reaction to the dream was to work harder. It was the one thing I knew how to do. We decided to put out more issues of the paper. We were up to doing six issues a year with 100,000 circulation in an area that included most of the central section of Missouri from Branson to Kirksville.

The part of the scene I could do nothing about, though, was the stuffing food in my mouth non-stop. The harder I worked, the more I wanted appreciation for my hard work. Meeting a deadline gave me a sense of accomplishment, quickly followed by the need to eat something to celebrate or reward myself. It was a cycle I couldn't break.

STORIES TRUMP DONUTS

I resigned myself to continuing to make God angry. Maybe I could work harder to make up for it. After all, I was doing what He had called me to do. It was affecting lives. Every issue brought praise reports from readers whose lives had been touched. Stories of lives changing kept me plugging away at publishing the newspaper. This was something I knew how to do. It was something I could do to make a difference. When I stood before God on judgment day and had to give account of everything I did, surely how many newspapers I published would trump how many donuts I had eaten. Wouldn't they?

Fast forward to 2013. I had just written about how compulsive overeating is an addiction and addiction is a sin. Somehow what I had written didn't feel good to me. I noticed a message a friend sent me about a scripture I had posted. He asked, "Would our conversation about grace be different these days versus last year? It sounds to me as if your position has moved." A year before he and I had an ongoing email discussion about works versus grace.

I told him I realized how in the past my emphasis on doing things for God had been a substitute for being connected in a deeper way with Him. But I still believed we were created for good works and they should be a part of who we are in Christ. I knew God would love me if I never did another thing. His grace was enough.

> I knew God would love me if I never did another thing.

I said, "If you are in Christ and the purpose is to do good works, then do them. I love my children no matter what they do, but when they pick up their clothes it makes me smile and when they don't it makes me frown."

I liked my answer. I thought I'd done a pretty good job of explaining the right position until I read his response: "God only frowns when we try to earn His smile, as that is pride which He always opposes."

His response was troublesome to me. I didn't want to answer him. I put it out of my mind. The next morning the minute I touched the floor of my prayer space I knew without a doubt God was leading me to change the way I communicated the message. I saw my whole approach of couching compulsive overeating as sin as not communicating God's heart. It was as if the fog lifted and I saw the message clearly.

GOD IS IN THE GRACE BUSINESS

So what if compulsive overeating, drinking, drugs, pornography and a million other things are sins? Jesus died for sin. God's grace covered all my sins. Remember grace? It's not just a girl's name. It's what God does. God is in the grace business.

God gives me grace so I can be the real me, the golden me, the me I have been hiding. The one I have been masking. The one I am afraid for others to see because it won't be good enough or awesome enough to make a difference.

When I was super morbidly obese I was always trying to earn God's favor by my works. Grace is God's unmerited favor. I already have it. Why did I, and do I still, try to earn it? Why did I spend long hours slaving, ignoring my family's needs and my own needs? What did I hope to gain?

The truth for me is compulsive overeating is a sin, but I also have the disease of sugar addiction. Where one starts and the other ends I'm not sure. For years, I understood compulsive overeating was not healthy, but I couldn't stop. The reason I couldn't stop was because my body had developed an addiction or sensitivity to sugar and gluten-causing grains. I knew gluttony was wrong, just like drunkenness was wrong[1] and I was into righting wrongs. I just couldn't right my own wrong.

WHAT GOD SAID

Some of what was wrong with me was an actual physical problem that had many layers to it. It took several doctors looking into what was happening with me to give me insights into how my body works and how I might start it in the right direction. Medical doctors, a fitness trainer, a physical therapist and a psychologist all recommended a sugar-free, gluten-free eating style. Had they been reading my prayer journals for the last 36 years?

God had been telling me to stop eating sugar all my adult life. Not listening to what He said was a sin. I did not listen even when I specifically asked Him to tell me how to lose weight.

I was accountable for what God instructed me to do.[2] I knew the right thing to do, but I just willfully chose not to do it, to turn my back on His suggestions. This started a harmful pattern I regret to this day.

I had the view that God was a slave driver cracking the whip rather than a benevolent leader concerned only for my best interests. The slave driver I saw wanted things done on time and perfectly. I couldn't do it. I assuaged the pressure and the guilt with food. It led to a downward spiral.

God showed me the throne room scene again. It was the same picture I'd seen before. The Father was on the throne. Jesus was at His right hand. The Holy Spirit was playing background music. I was down below at my highest weight. This time, though, I saw some things I hadn't seen before.

The Father and the Son's heads were together in what I had thought was a conferring posture. On closer examination I clearly saw there were tears in their eyes. The music the Holy Spirit was playing was not angry like a howling wind, but mournful.

God was not mad, He was sad. He was sad because of all the obstacles I had put in my path to reach the abundance He had for me. He was sad because I might never reach the potential He placed inside me. He was sad because I clearly loved food more than I loved Him.

And yet, in His power and wisdom, He gave me more grace.[3] Grace I learned was not just some power by which we receive salvation.[4] Grace is power, energy, fluid movement, unforced rhythm, persistence and patience.

EMPLOYING GRACE

The power of grace is a lot like an engine. It only started really activating in my life when I took the first step and began exercising and eating right. When I did that, His grace propelled me forward towards exercise like a whirlwind. His grace ate up my desire for unhealthy food like a wildfire. Dancing to the unforced rhythms of grace definitely set my life on fire.

Brash, excitable Peter encouraged us to employ grace. He was older and wiser when he wrote about grace. "Each of you has received a gift (a particular spiritual talent, a gracious divine endowment), employ it for one another as [befits] good trustees of God's many-sided grace [faithful stewards of the extremely diverse powers and gifts granted to Christians by unmerited favor]."[5]

The word "employ," according to the dictionary, means to make use of. So how do I make use of grace? And if grace is the power of God, the fluid movement of God, what could employing it to its full potential do for me, my family, my church and my community? Beyond that, what could power, favor and blessing in my life do for the kingdom of God?

Grace is the heavenly part of the equation that blows everything to exponential proportions. It is the operating system that works in the background of my life, but only comes alive when I hit the start button.

Peter knew what grace was all about. He, maybe more than all the disciples, experienced God's grace in the form of forgiveness. It was the grace of forgiveness that captured his heart and propelled him to see that by employing the other aspects of the grace, he and his fellow disciples could access all the fullness of God. They, together with grace, were able to do the impossible.

He understood if God's people really employed the many-sided benefits of grace, the multitudes could be brought into God's Kingdom. The main purpose of grace is not for me to spend cheaply, squandering it on my wants and desires. Grace is for me to employ to accomplish the kingdom of God on the earth. That gives my life meaning and purpose. It makes me want to follow His ways all my life.

UNFORCED RHYTHMS OF GRACE

Walking in His ways, following after meaning and purpose, happens as I dare to believe that the power of His grace is movement that flows through me to the world. When I push start and agree to cooperate with God, the unforced rhythms of grace take over.

Grace is why I'm here. It's what keeps me going even when I do something ridiculous that looks like I'm thumbing my nose at God, such as eating whatever I want. Grace draws me back. As I repent, God dusts me off and points me in the right direction, reminding me when I veer off my chosen path that I'm going the wrong way. He clearly leads me to the paths of righteousness.

God's grace always draws me back when I fall.

It's a fluid motion that causes me to be swept along. God's grace delivers gifts to make my movement here on earth almost effortless. And when things crash to the ground, it's God's grace that gently picks me up.

I can't imagine living this life without the unfathomable depths of the grace of an all-powerful God. Dancing to the unforced rhythms of grace cannot help but set my life on fire.

ENDNOTES

1. Ezekiel 16:49, Deuteronomy 21:20, Proverbs 23:21, Proverbs 23:2, Matthew 23:25, NKJV; Galatians 5:19-21, Weymouth New Testament.
2. James 4:17, NIV
3. James 4:6, NIV
4. Ephesians 2:8-9, NIV
5. 1 Peter 4:10, AMP

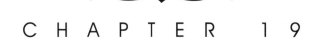

C H A P T E R   1 9

FORGIVE

"Bear with each other and forgive whatever grievances you may have against one another. Forgive as the Lord forgave you."

Colossians 3:13, NIV

I was doing a Bible study on forgiveness. It suggested writing a letter to the person you need to forgive. The study said sending it was not necessary, just the act of writing it saying I forgive the person for whatever issue would be enough.

I had not realized I needed to forgive my mother. I figured what happened when I was a child, happened. She was sick and could not help what she did or didn't do.

Stuffing my feelings, though, was not working for me. At this time, she was really physically sick. She had colon cancer. I was having a hard time feeling any emotion over her illness. So I took the suggestion and wrote the letter and forgave her for not being there when I was a child, for putting too much responsibility on me at such a young age, for her extreme rage and unrealistic punishment of me as a child. I wrote the letter and then tore it up. It was extremely freeing.

Some areas of forgiveness take more time and effort. Forgiving Fred was a one time thing I did during a sermon. A woman was speaking about her journey through a living hell being sexually abused by her father. Before that Fred loomed larger than life in my mind even though he was deceased. After I forgave him, he appeared as a shriveled up old man. I saw myself as an 11-year old girl sit up in that bed and scream. He fled never to return, the door slamming shut as he left.

I still had the wall of protection in place in my life. Removing that took conscious determination and realization that God as my Father did, will and continues to protect me.

Forgiveness is a command. Jesus said, "For if you forgive men when they sin against you, your heavenly Father will also forgive you. But if you do not forgive men their sins, your Father will not forgive your sins."[1]

Someone told me I really didn't forgive my mother because I didn't talk to her face-to-face. Forgiveness is a choice. I didn't need her recognition of the offenses. Much of what I went through was how I perceived and processed what happened. She did not need to know all the ways I felt hurt. I know she did not knowingly decide she was going to do some of the things she did. I did not want or need justice. I only wanted to be free of the feelings I had.

Only God can bring freedom, but He can't do it if I don't forgive. Joyfully I forgave her. Then I could begin to feel for and with her. In the months leading up to her funeral, I cried years of tears for her. Sitting by her bedside, we bonded in ways we hadn't really done before. At her funeral, my sorrow was genuine.

HOW MANY TIMES?

Peter asked Jesus a question about how many times it is necessary to forgive. Most remember the answer. He said seven times seventy, which to me means an infinite number of times or continually forgiving. After He gives Peter the answer, He explains it with a parable.[2]

Let me summarize and paraphrase. A guy owes the king like a million dollars. The king was going to throw him in jail but he begged to be allowed to pay it back. Instead, the king totally erased the debt.

No sooner had he left the king than he saw an acquaintance that owed him ten dollars. He demanded payment. The acquaintance begged for mercy. Instead of extending the same treatment the king had given him, he threw the guy who owed him 10 bucks in jail.

The king was quite angry and threw the first guy in jail because he had not shown mercy to the acquaintance. The king put him in jail until he could pay back the debt. Of course the man could never repay the debt.

Looking at the story, I see the three characters are the king, the guy and his acquaintance. The king is God. The guy is me. His acquaintance is the person who wronged me.

In the last verse God says if we don't forgive the acquaintance, He will put us in jail.[3] I don't want to be in jail. It denotes not being able to do anything or accomplish anything. To me, it is akin to spinning your wheels.

If I don't forgive, bitterness over what was done to me will eventually block me from moving forward to wholeness and healing. The offense leads me to want to protect myself or make myself bigger in order to handle situations that are thrown at me until I forgive the person.

Forgiveness brings inner healing. Forgiveness helps me understand that my desire to be physically healthy is not just a whim. It is a permanent decision.

Forgiveness brings inner healing.

My unhealthy lifestyle is not something I will run back to when I am in situations for which I feel unprepared or ill-equipped.

Recently I went on a different kind of journey, a prayer and inner healing journey towards seeing and understanding how many issues in my past that still affect my future. I had to once again do some forgiving for things that came up in researching my past. This journey was spiritual in every way. What follows is a part of this experience.

WHOLENESS

My mother's foot is in the door of fear I'm trying to shut. I don't want it there. It's keeping the door open for hurts, disappointments and rejection.

It seems so much of me is wrapped up in trying to figure her out, even though she is gone and I'm not a child anymore. Still

I contemplate and extend so much energy, even unconsciously towards her.

She feels bigger than life to me, bigger than God. Even when I slam the door, I worry she will push against it relentlessly until it opens a crack and my feelings of fear, mistrust and confusion flood back in.

Releasing the pain from my life is the only way to freedom, the only way to become totally and completely me. Because forgiveness is a process, I forgive her again for many things, but mostly for not comforting me as a child in the way I needed to be comforted. Because of that I sometimes feel the Holy Spirit will not comfort me. This is a lie.

The truth is He is my comforter and the only One who can and does comfort me. I feel the breath of Him inside filling me up so much it crowds out the need for comfort foods, which only make me even more uncomfortable.

I check cautiously to see the disposition of the door. It stays shut sealed by the blood of Jesus and finally I know God is bigger, stronger than anyone, even my mother, even the man who would abuse me, even my childhood fears.

WALL OF PROTECTION

Once the door is shut, though, I must deal with my wall of protection, the one I hide behind, the one that supposedly keeps me safe. I want to keep it in place. I don't want to give it up and yet it's keeping me from the good things, the gold and the abundance.

I see it clearly now. It looks much like a two-foot thick chocolate armor shell entrapping me. Chocolate should not be hard to break, but this won't budge. It's stuck to me. I see no way to remove it without removing part of me.

I ask Father God what I should use to remove this barrier I have created. Even though I have lost weight, I know emotionally and spiritually the shell still exists. I need to be whole in every area. I need to have no obstacles between Father God and myself.

There is still part of me that believes I may need the physical wall of flesh back one day. There may be someone who overwhelms, controls and manipulates me. I may want to hide inside my sugarcoated tomb again.

Removal of the shell is beyond my comprehension until He hands me a huge bucket of water. I look at the bucket and back into His eyes. He doesn't say a word, but I instantly know I am to pour the bucket over myself. When I do the hard, thick sugary shell melts. Along with it my need for self-protection dissolves.

> Though I can blame others for what has happened to me, I cannot hold on to that for it will ruin me.

I am truly free to feel the comfort of the Holy Spirit, the love of Father God and the companionship of Jesus. I run to the lap of Father God. He holds, loves, protects and supports me. And tells me I am beautiful. I am creative. I am destined for abundance. I believe Him because He is not only my Father; He is my perfect Mother, my Best Friend.

I was broken by things in my past. Some things are difficult to define and though I can blame others for what has happened to me, I cannot hold on to that for it will ruin me. I forgive, again and again bringing wholeness with each breath, each breaking of the past.

EMBRACE THE GOLD

To move forward I must accept and embrace the gold within me. That gold or worth and value used to frighten me. It overwhelmed and threatened to get ahead of me, overtake me and consume me. I wanted to cover it up, squelch it so people wouldn't expect too much of me.

I was so afraid of letting the gold shine. Hiding the gold so no one but me knew about it helped me relax a little. If my performance didn't produce what I wanted then I wasn't letting anyone down, but me.

In fact, hiding the gold let myself and everyone else down. Why would God give me gifts if He didn't want me to use them? Letting go of all the hers and hims who damaged, threatened, taunted, cursed and undid me, released me to grab hold of everything that is right, true, honorable, just and excitingly new in my life.

Gifts were given for me to release into God's perfect care. I do not have to strive or perform perfectly. I can cease from performance and give all to Him who will multiply even the smallest things for His glory.

I am saved. I am healed. I am delivered. I walk in freedom and wholeness. Ah yes, wholeness, what I crave, what I desire. I want to be complete in Him and complete in myself, to accept all the good things God has for me.

I shut the door to the difficulties in the past. There is no possibility of it opening as it is sealed closed. I renounce the lies that Father God does not care about me and embrace the truth that He fights for me, protects me and loves me so very much.

Now I can see the gold before me, unlimited opportunity, unlimited potential in God. I can rest and allow the gold to shine as only gold can when polished by Creator God.

ENDNOTES

1. Matthew 6:14-15, NIV
2. Matthew 18:23-35, NIV
3. Matthew 18:25, NIV

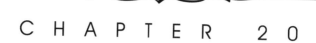

CHAPTER 20

ABUNDANCE

"I have come that you might have life—
life in all its fullness."

John 10:10b, GNB

The journey through super morbid obesity can only be likened to a trip to hell and back again. No matter how difficult the trip, though, it is life-changing in ways I could never have imagined.

For me it is, and has been, a journey of highs and lows, of despair and ecstasy, of pain and relief. Most of all, though, the journey has been one of willful self-indulgence and physical desires.

The journey back was harder than the journey there because it involved pain and sacrifice. It involved giving up what I thought was bringing me comfort, only to clearly see they were leading to a sure and certain early death. I was committing suicide slowly, sweet morsel by sweet morsel. These sugary substances are poison to me. Most of the rest of the world enjoys these delicacies in moderation, but I cannot because I can't just stop with one.

Now I see the possibility of being victorious in this life-long battle with sugar. It almost took me under. It almost took my life. In many ways it did take some of the best years of my life when my children were growing up and when I could have had more impact with my ministry.

There are times when the goal was so close I could touch it, taste it and feel it. And there were times when I wondered, "What will happen next?" "What will I give in to?" "Why am I so weak?" "Why can I not just be normal all by myself?" "Will I be able to resist temptation for the rest of my life?"

And then I remember what giving in to this disease called sugar addiction did to me. I remember the scale-tipping weight. I remember regretting eating the first piece of candy. God's grace for all my addiction to sweets showered over me in forgiveness when I recognized and turned away from it. When I allowed Him to, His sweet grace became a vehicle of power to help me do what I always thought impossible. It took me to turn the key, to take the first step, to begin. Once beginning, I found God's sweet grace was there all along if only I had taken hold of it by my actions. Because I have listened to the call of grace, I have good strategies and boundaries and plans in place. It is God's plan that promises to prosper me with a hope and a future. And He always keeps His promises.

I finally agreed with God and He helped me stop the progression that would end in my death. But my indulgences had their consequences.

I may have permanently damaged my joints by carrying more than 250 pounds of excess weight. I can't walk long distances or run. One day, I will walk and leap and praise God while I'm doing it. Today may be the day, but if not here, I know it will happen in the land to come.

Since I decided to have weight loss surgery in the process, I have to take a cabinet full of vitamins and minerals because my system does not absorb minerals readily.

I need to be on guard at all times lest the enemy tempt me with sweets shaped like a caramel saying, "Just this one time won't matter. After all, you are smart. You can control yourself." And that is a lie from the pit of hell. I cannot control myself. I acknowledge I am powerless over food, that I need a Power greater than myself to restore me to sanity, and that I turn the control of my life completely over to God. This was not a one-time decision. It is a moment-by-moment choice.

MASTER CONNECTION

The most beautiful part of the return journey, no matter how treacherous, is the close communion with the Master. There is a definite sweetness that comes in admitting I have an area of my life that is out of control. When I turn that over to God, not to magically remove the weight, but to walk with me as I look to Him for guidance every step of the way, I experience more grace. His grace covers me every time I slip down a sticky slope instead of asking for His guidance. His grace draws me back to Him time and time again. As I repent, He forgives me completely, no matter what I do.

He has grace for sugar addiction. He has grace for how I damaged my body, His temple. He has grace for me because He loves me. His sweet grace, always leads me straight to Him.

- I experienced shame. He gave me
  more than enough grace.

- I experienced withdrawal. He
  reminded me of His presence.

- I experienced regret. He gave me redemption.

- I experienced confusion. He gave me peace.

- I experienced pride. He gave me humility.

- I experienced impatience. He gave me patience.

- I experienced depression. He gave me joy.

- I experienced loneliness. He gave me love.

- I experienced being totally unable to control my
  wants and desires. He gave me self-control by
  placing His Spirit inside me to gently remind me
  it is possible to be so totally sold out to Him that
  it will override my craving for sugar and bread.

GOD IS ALREADY THERE

Everything I need God already has provided. Wherever I am, God is already there. I don't have to conjure Him up with certain scriptures or prayers or behaviors. He's already there in each and every moment of my life.

He longs to be involved, but only at the point of my honest and open transparency before Him. He won't physically remove the donut from my hand, but He will, at my invitation, remind me of my former decision. If I start listening and obeying, He will keep reminding me. When I forget or don't listen, He will stop. If I come back and lay it all before Him, He will be there to patiently and gently guide me forward, reminding me of His supernatural purpose for my natural body here today.

I may think God has it in for me because I have a natural inclination towards sugar. Others can eat sweets and not gain an ounce because sugar does not propel them towards obsession. I eat sugar and can't stop, thereby gaining the weight of two people. I cry out to God, "Why me?"

Here's the truth of the matter. God loves me so much He specifically designed me with a weakness that keeps me dependent on Him for any measure of success. For the rest of my life I will know I have a weakness which can only be met by throwing open the doors to my secret candy stash and allowing Him to see every time I have eaten to excess and every time I want to do it so badly I can taste the desire. Yet, His strength is made perfect in my weakness. And He meets me there with open arms.

I NEED GOD MORE THAN SUGAR

I have cried out to God as I thought back through the years and realized what I did to myself, my family, my friends and my God. The process of revisiting what I did was not easy, but in the final analysis I learned one overwhelming thing: I need God more than sugar.

I need Him to show me how to do the very basic things, like how to eat, how to love, how to give and how to humble myself. I don't need to ask Him if I should eat healthy or exercise. I already know He wants me to do that.

I do need Him to walk with me as I make decisions one step at a time. And when I turn the wrong way, I need Him to be that voice behind me that says, "No, this is the walk. Walk here."[1] And, I will. I will turn away when I am headed in the wrong direction that leads me back down deadly pathways.

I will turn towards healthy foods like fresh vegetables, fresh fruits and lean protein. I will turn away from sugar, breads and starches. I will turn towards clean, pure water. I will turn away from my desire for sodas. I will turn towards movement of some kind, any kind, even if it is just a walk around the block. I will turn away from sitting and vegetating mindlessly watching a television show I've already seen three times.

I will do these things because I am sick. And I am tired. My life has become unmanageable and I hate being out of control.

HEAVENLY CHEERLEADERS

God knows all about everything in my past. He was there. He's here now, right by my side rooting for me all the way. But He's not the only one. Friends, family and those who don't even know me have supported me, encouraged me, loved me, and lifted me up.

Some of my biggest encouragers, who have gone on before me, also see me and are rooting for me not only to finish, but to finish well. That propels me towards my goal of being all God wants me to be. I hear the crowds cheering for me as I tackle this great task with the Holy Spirit's help.

"Since I am surrounded by so great a crowd of witnesses, I will lay aside the unnecessary weight and the compulsive overeating which so easily clings to and entangles me. I will run the appointed race that is set before me with patient endurance, being steady and having active persistence.

"Looking away from every delectable morsel of food that distracts me from my appointed course of action to Jesus, the One who demonstrated how to live in the world and will help me finish this appointed course of action with maturity and perfection.

"So right now, I will invigorate myself. I lift up my drooping hands. I will strengthen my feeble and tottering knees. I will make a firm, plain, smooth, straight path for my feet. I will set my face toward a path of happiness going in the right direction. This path of health and vigor will help my lame and halting limbs so they are not put out of joint, but are cured."[2]

It is only by seeing the journey for what it is, a life-changing journey for the rest of my natural days that I am victorious.

I can never go back to my old ways. The old ways are dead to me. I am a new person.[3] I have new ways of coping with the world, new ways of looking at life. My old life is gone. I buried it in the same box I used to put myself in when I was working to please God. Today, I don't have to think about the old life, only the new one, only the better way I have chosen.

> I have new ways of coping with the world, new ways of looking at life.

I am not on this journey to arrive somewhere. I am on this journey to be the best, most vibrant and healthy me possible. I am on this journey to cooperate with the Master to get to know Him better.

I am not on this journey to please someone else, to become someone else or to call attention to myself. I am on this journey to discover more of the divine spark that God has placed inside of me.

I do not have to berate myself or beat myself up for past failures or demises my compulsive overeating may have caused in relationships, jobs or dreams.

DEPTHS OF GOD'S GRACE

I am on this journey to discover the depths of God's grace. It is a grace He provided to bring me to Himself. It is a grace He provides to cover my weakness. It is a grace that grows throughout eternity. I did nothing to earn it. I can do nothing to keep it. It is God's divine unmerited favor and blessing that pervades every pore of my being and every minute of my life.

His grace has movement. It is because of His grace that I flow with Him and become more of who I am called to be. It is because of His grace I can leap tall mountains of flesh in a single moment of decision. It is because of His grace I am no longer bound by sugary chains of weakness. His grace has power to propel me towards His goal for me, but only if I'm moving first, only if I'm acknowledging the need for his supernatural grace in my life.

> It is because of His grace I am no longer bound by sugary chains of weakness.

I have all that I need to succeed. I am "self-sufficient in Christ's sufficiency"[4] of grace. I know beyond a shadow of a doubt that I have power to go forward and accomplish the task because His power is made perfect in my weakness.[5]

Without His grace I would be close to death's door. Instead, I am standing surrounded by His favor and blessing.

He rescued me from the pit. He showed me the steps I need to take to come out of bondage. I am not alone.

He has been walking with me every step on this journey, and now I am swimming in the power-filled abundance of His sweet grace.

ENDNOTES

1. Isaiah 30:21, NIV
2. Paraphrased from Hebrews 12:1-2, 12-13, AMP
3. 2 Corinthians 5:17, NIV
4. Philippians 4:13, AMP
5. 2 Corinthians 12:9, NIV

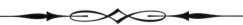

FINAL NOTE

"You keep track of all my sorrows. You have collected all my tears in your bottle. You have recorded each one in your book."

Psalm 56:8, NLT

I can't end without sharing a letter my daughter, who is teaching English in Japan, wrote regarding my lifelong struggle with food. I invited her to tell me how having a morbidly obese mother affected her. As you read this letter, please think of those near and dear to you.

- What kind of impact will your difficulties have on them? How can you change a negative into a positive?

- Is it worth the effort?

I'll let Jenny's letter answer that question for you.

Dear Mom,

I don't remember being embarrassed by your size. I'm sure the bullies in my elementary school probably used it as ammunition, but they'd use anything. Regardless, I wasn't embarrassed by your size. I could care less about how you looked. You're my mom and I love you.

I do remember regretting how much time you spent working. Remember when your desk was in the living room? I wanted to play; I wanted to spend time with you. You told me, "This is an office. This is a place of work." And I went to my room and cried because if I couldn't call the living room home, then where could I call home? I dreamed silly little girl dreams of living in a world where no one ever had to work and everywhere was home.

I do remember you getting angry, especially with Andrew for not doing something or another that you told him to do. Whenever you got mad at me, I internalized it, even if I was passive aggressive about it or talked back, I still internalized it. I had done something wrong and I should change. But when it happened to Andrew, because he was so good, I felt it was unprovoked. He didn't deserve it. It's an odd feeling for a little girl to want to protect her older brother from her mother. It's really strange to feel that sort of responsibility at such a young age, but then you've felt that more than I ever had to.

I remember feeling at home because hugging you felt like hugging a big warm pillow. And I do mean that as a compliment.

I remember feeling a bit of resentment because you'd have me do the most menial things for you because you didn't even want to get up and walk to the kitchen to do it yourself.

It was different after you had your knee surgery. It was the same menial tasks I had resented as a child: "Get me something to eat from the kitchen." "Grab this from my desk." "Go get my purse." But I didn't resent it any more. I had more respect for you, because you were constantly trying to be a better person.

You haven't given up, and that's truly awe-inspiring. When I read about the research on morbid obesity, there's a lot to support that it is passed down through the generations. I can't deny the fact I was raised by a morbidly obese mother, but you've beaten those statistics. And I know that you will always get back up again.

You've mentioned a time that you were gaining weight after your bypass surgery, but I don't remember it because I had faith you would lose the weight and be healthy again.

I watched you battle with your own demons for years. You've inspired so many people. You continue to inspire me. I'm proud of you, Mom. I can't wait until everyone can read your story and be inspired as well.

—Jenny Parker
Ichinoseki-shi, Japan

OK, I'm crying now. Go out and change your world. Start with you. You can do it. I believe in you. Go be awesome.

SCRIPTURES

PROLOGUE

Romans 7:24, AMP. *"Oh unhappy and pitiable and wretched woman that I am, who will release and deliver me from [the shackles of] this body of death?"*

Ephesians 1:7b-8, CEB. *"We have forgiveness for our failures based on His overflowing grace, which He poured over us with wisdom and understanding."*

CHAPTER 1

Ephesians 2:8-9, NIV. *"For it is by grace you have been saved, through faith—and this is not from yourselves, it is the gift of God—not by works, so that no one can boast."*

CHAPTER 2

Dueteronomy 30:19-20, NLT. *"Today I have given you the choice between life and death, between blessings and curses. I call on heaven and earth to witness the choice you make. Oh, that you would choose life, that you and your descendants might live! Choose to love the Lord your God and to obey Him and commit yourself to Him, for He is your life. Then you will live long in the land the Lord swore to give your ancestors Abraham, Isaac, and Jacob."*

Matthew 17:20, NIV. *"He replied, 'Because you have so little faith. Truly I tell you, if you have faith as small as a mustard* seed, you can say to this mountain, 'Move from here to there,' and it will move. Nothing will be impossible for you.'"

CHAPTER 3

1 Corintians 13:12, NLT. *"Now we see things imperfectly, like puzzling reflections in a mirror, but then we will see everything with perfect clarity. All that I know now is partial and incomplete, but then I will know everything completely, just as God now knows me completely."*

CHAPTER 4

Romans 3:23-24, NIV. *"For all have sinned and fall short of the glory of God and are justified freely by His grace through the redemption that came by Christ Jesus."*

CHAPTER 5

Proverbs 25:28, NIV. *"Like a city whose walls are broken through is a person who lacks self-control."*

Galatians 5:19-21, Weymouth New Testament. *"Now you know full well the doings of our lower natures. Fornication, impurity, indecency, idol-worship, sorcery; enmity, strife, jealousy, outbursts of passion, intrigues, dissensions, factions, envyings; hard drinking, riotous feasting, and the like. And as to these I forewarn you, as I have already forewarned you, that those who are guilty of such things will have no share in the Kingdom of God."*

CHAPTER 6

Proverbs 3:5-8, MSG. *"Trust God from the bottom of your heart; don't try to figure out everything on your own. Listen* *for God's voice in everything you do, everywhere you go; He's the One who will keep you on track. Don't assume that you know it all. Run to God. Run from evil. Your body will glow with health, your very bones will vibrate with life."*

Ephesians 3:20, NIV. *"Now to Him who is able to do immeasurably more than all we ask or imagine, according to his power that is at work within us."*

CHAPTER 7

1 Corinthians 13:11, NLT. *"When I was a child, I talked like a child, I spoke and thought and reasoned as a child. But when I grew up, I put away childish things."*

1 Timothy 4:2, NIV. *"Such teachings come through hypocritical liars, whose consciences have been seared as with a hot iron."*

CHAPTER 8

1 Corinthians 13:4-8, NLT. *"Love is patient and kind. Love is not jealous or boastful or proud or rude. Love does not demand its own way. Love is not irritable, and it keeps no record of when it has been wronged. It is never glad about injustice but rejoices whenever the truth wins out. Love never gives up, never loses faith, is always hopeful, and endures through every circumstance. Love will last forever."*

James 4:17, NIV. *"If anyone, then, knows the good they ought to do and doesn't do it, it is sin for them."*

Psalm 78: 18, 25, NIV. *"They willfully put God to the test by demanding the food they craved ... They ate the bread of angels; He sent them all the food they could eat."*

Ephesians 5:25, NIV. *"Husbands, love your wives, just as Christ loved the church and gave himself up for her."*

CHAPTER 9

Psalm 34:7-8, NIV. *"The angel of the Lord encamps around those who fear Him, and He delivers them. Taste and see that the Lord is good ; blessed is the man who takes refuge in Him."*

Isaiah 66:1, NIV. *"This is what the Lord says: 'Heaven is my throne, and the earth is my footstool.'"*

Proverbs 31:30, AMP. *"Charm and grace are deceptive, and beauty is vain [because it is not lasting], but a woman who reverently and worshipfully fears the Lord, she shall be praised!"*

Proverbs 1:7, NIV. *"The fear of the Lord is the beginning of knowledge, but fools despise wisdom and instruction."*

Proverbs 9:10, NIV. *"The fear of the Lord is the beginning of wisdom, and knowledge of the Holy One is understanding."*

1 John 4:18, NKJV. *"There is no fear in love; but perfect love casts out fear, because fear involves torment. But he who fears has not been made perfect in love."*

Psalm 139: 13-16, NIV. *"For you created my inmost being; You knit me together in my mother's womb. I praise You because I am fearfully and wonderfully made; Your works are wonderful, I know that full well. My frame was not hidden from You when I was made in the secret place, when I was woven together in the depths of the earth. Your eyes saw my unformed body; all the days ordained for me were written in Your book before one of them came to be."*

Matthew 5:6, NIV. *"Blessed are those who hunger and thirst for righteousness, for they will be filled."*

John 4:33, NLT. *"'Did someone bring Him food while* **we were** *gone?' the disciples asked each other."*

CHAPTER 10

John 8:32, NKJV. *"And you shall know the truth, and the truth will set you free."*

CHAPTER 11

Genesis 25:30-32, NLT. *"Esau said to Jacob, 'I'm starved. Give me some of that red stew.' 'All right,' Jacob replied, 'but trade me your rights as the firstborn son.' 'Look, I'm dying of starvation,' said Esau. 'What good is my birthright to me now?'"*

Hebrews 4:16, NIV. *"Let us then approach God's throne of grace with confidence, so that we may receive mercy and find grace to help us in our time of need."*

Ephesians 1:3, NIV. *"Praise be to the God and Father of our Lord Jesus Christ, who has blessed us in the heavenly realms with every spiritual blessing in Christ."*

Matthew 7:9-11, NIV. *"Which of you, if your son asks for bread, will give him a stone? Or if he asks for a fish, will give him a snake? If you, then, though you are evil, know how to give good gifts to your children, how much more will your Father in heaven give good gifts to those who ask Him!"*

Psalm 42:5, NIV. *"Why, my soul, are you downcast? Why so disturbed within me? Put your hope in God, for I will yet praise Him, my Savior and my God."*

Hebrews 4:15, NIV. *"For we do not have a high priest who is unable to empathize with our weaknesses, but we have One who has been tempted in every way, just as we are—yet He did not sin."*

Romans 7:15-24, NIV. *"I do not understand what I do. For what I want to do I do not do, but what I hate I do. And if I do what I do not want to do, I agree that the law is good. As it is, it is no longer I myself who do it, but it is sin living in me. For I know that good itself does not dwell in me, that is, in my sinful nature. For I have the desire to do what is good, but I cannot carry it out. For I do not do the good I want to do, but the evil I do not want to do—this I keep on doing. Now if I do what I do not want to do, it is no longer I who do it, but it is sin living in me that does it. So I find this law at work: although I want to do good, evil is right there with me. For in my inner being I delight in God's law; but I see another law at work in me, waging war against the law of my mind and making me a prisoner of the law of sin at work within me. What a wretched man I am! Who will rescue me from this body that is subject to death?"*

James 4:6, NIV. *"But He gives us more grace. That is why Scripture says: 'God opposes the proud, but shows favor to the humble.'"*

James 4:7, NIV. *"Submit yourselves, then, to God. Resist the devil, and he will flee from you."*

CHAPTER 12

Acts 12:7, NASB. *"And behold, an angel of the Lord suddenly appeared and a light shone in the cell; and he struck Peter's side and woke him up, saying, 'Get up quickly.' And his chains fell off his hands."*

CHAPTER 13

Philippians 3:18-20, NIV. *"For, as I have often told you before and now tell you again even with tears, many live as enemies of the cross of Christ. Their destiny is destruction, their god is their stomach, and their glory is in their shame. Their mind is set on earthly things. But our citizenship is in heaven."*

CHAPTER 14

1 Corinthians 6:12, NASB. *"All things are lawful for me, but not all things are profitable. All things are lawful for me, but I will not be mastered by anything."*

CHAPTER 15

3 John 2, NKJV. *"Beloved, I pray that you may prosper in all things and be in health, just as your soul prospers."*

Ephesians 2:3, NIV. *"All of us also lived among them at one time, gratifying the cravings of our flesh and following its desires and thoughts. Like the rest, we were by nature deserving of wrath."*

Isaiah 30:21, NIV. *"Whether you turn to the right or to the left, your ears will hear a voice behind you, saying, 'This is the way; walk in it.'"*

Matthew 25:24-28, NIV. *"Then the man who had received one bag of gold came. 'Master,' he said, 'I knew that you are a hard man, harvesting where you have not sown and gathering where you have not scattered seed. So I was afraid and went out and hid your gold in the ground. See, here is what belongs to you.' His master replied, 'You wicked, lazy servant! So you knew that I harvest where I have not sown and gather where I have not scattered seed? Well then, you should have put my money on deposit with the bankers, so that when I returned I would have received it back with interest.'"*

Galatians 5:22-23, NIV. *"But the fruit of the Spirit is love, joy, peace, forbearance, kindness, goodness, faithfulness, gentleness and self-control. Against such things there is no law."*

Ephesians 5:29. NKJV. *"For no one ever hated his own flesh, but nourishes and cherishes it, just as the Lord does the church."*

2 Corinthians 12:9-10, NIV. *"But He said to me, 'My grace is sufficient for you, for My power is made perfect in weakness.' Therefore I will boast all the more gladly about my weaknesses, so that Christ's power may rest on me. That is why, for Christ's sake, I delight in weaknesses, in insults, in hardships, in persecutions, in difficulties. For when I am weak, then I am strong."*

CHAPTER 16

1 Corinthians 10:13, NET. *"No trial has overtaken you that is not faced by others. And God is faithful: He will not let you be tried beyond what you are able to bear, but with the trial will also provide a way out so that you may be able to endure it."*

John 10:10, NIV. *"The thief comes only to steal and kill and destroy; I have come that they may have life, and have it to the full."*

Romans 8:11, NIRV. *"The Spirit of the One who raised Jesus from the dead is living in you. So the God who raised Christ from the dead will also give life to your bodies, which are going to die. He will do this by the power of His Spirit, who lives in you."*

Isaiah 50:7, NIV. *"Because the Sovereign Lord helps me, I will not be disgraced. Therefore have I set my face like flint, and I know I will not be put to shame."*

CHAPTER 17

Ephesians 3:20, MSG. *"God can do anything, you know— far more than you could ever imagine or guess or request in your wildest dreams! He does it not by pushing us around but by working within us, His Spirit deeply and gently within us."*

CHAPTER 18

Ezekiel 16:49, NKJV. *"Look, this was the iniquity of your sister Sodom: She and her daughter had pride, fullness of food, and abundance of idleness; neither did she strengthen the hand of the poor and needy."*

Deuteronomy 21:20, NKJV. *"And they shall say to the elders of his city, 'This son of ours is stubborn and rebellious; he will not obey our voice; he is a glutton and a drunkard.'"*

Proverbs 23:21, NKJV. *"For the drunkard and the glutton will come to poverty, And drowsiness will clothe a man with rags."*

Proverbs 23:2, NKJV. *"And put a knife to your throat if you are a man given to appetite."*

Matthew 23:25, NKJV. *"Woe to you, scribes and Pharisees, hypocrites! For you cleanse the outside of the cup and dish, but inside they are full of extortion and self-indulgence."*

1 Peter 4:10, AMP. *"As each of you has received a gift (a particular spiritual talent, a gracious divine endowment), employ it for one another as [befits] good trustees of God's many-sided grace [faithful stewards of the extremely diverse powers and gifts granted to Christians by unmerited favor]."*

Colossians 3:13, NIV. *"Bear with each other and forgive one another if any of you has a grievance against someone. Forgive as the Lord forgave you."*

Matthew 6:14-15, NIV. *"For if you forgive other people when they sin against you, your heavenly Father will also forgive you. But if you do not forgive others their sins, your Father will not forgive your sins."*

Matthew 18: 23-35, NIV. *"Therefore, the kingdom of heaven is like a king who wanted to settle accounts with his servants. As he began the settlement, a man who owed him ten thousand bags of gold was brought to him. Since he was not able to pay, the master ordered that he and his wife and his children and all that he had be sold to repay the debt. At this the servant fell on his knees before him. 'Be patient with me,' he begged, 'and I will pay back everything.' The servant's master took pity on him, canceled the debt and let him go. But when that servant went out, he found one of his fellow servants who owed him a hundred silver coins. He grabbed him and began to choke him. 'Pay back what you owe me!' he demanded. His fellow servant* *fell to his knees and begged him, 'Be patient with me, and I will pay it back.' But he refused. Instead, he went off and had the man thrown into prison until he could pay the debt. When the other servants saw what had happened, they were outraged and went and told their master everything that had happened. Then the master called the servant in. 'You wicked servant,' he said, 'I canceled all that debt of yours because you begged me to. Shouldn't you have had mercy on your fellow servant just as I had on you?' In anger his master handed him over to the jailers to be tortured, until he should pay back all he owed. This is how my heavenly Father will treat each of you unless you forgive your brother or sister from your heart."*

CHAPTER 20

John 10:10b, GNB. *"I have come that you might have life—life in all its fullness."*

Hebrews 12:1-2, 12-13, AMP. *"Therefore then, since we are surrounded by so great a cloud of witnesses [who have borne testimony to the Truth], let us strip off and throw aside every encumbrance (unnecessary weight) and that sin which so readily (deftly and cleverly) clings to and entangles us, and let us run with patient endurance and steady and active persistence the appointed course of the race that is set before us, looking away [from all that will distract] to Jesus, Who is the Leader and the Source of our faith [giving the first incentive for our belief] and is also its Finisher [bringing it to maturity and perfection]. He, for the joy [of obtaining the prize] that was set before Him, endured the cross, despising and ignoring the shame, and is now seated at the right hand of the throne of God.*

2 Corinthians 5:17, NIV. *"Therefore, if anyone is in Christ, the new creation has come: the old has gone, the new is here!"*

Philippians 4:13, AMP. *"I have strength for all things in Christ Who empowers me [I am ready for anything and equal to anything through Him Who infuses inner strength into me; I am self-sufficient in Christ's sufficiency]."*

CHAPTER 21

Jeremiah 29:11, NIV. *"'For I know the plans I have for you,' declares the Lord, 'plans to prosper you and not to harm you, plans to give you hope and a future.'"*

EPILOGUE

Zephaniah 3:17, NLT. *"For the Lord your God is living among you. He is a mighty Savior. He will take delight in you with gladness. With His love, He will calm all your fears. He will rejoice over you with joyful songs."*

FINAL NOTE

Psalm 56:8, NLT. *"You keep track of all my sorrows. You have collected all my tears in your bottle. You have recorded each one in your book."*

TERESA SHIELDS PARKER
BEFORE & AFTER

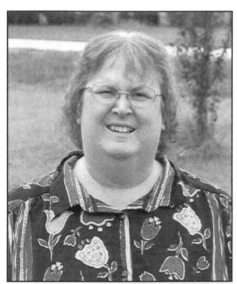
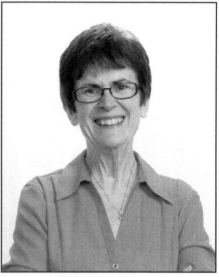
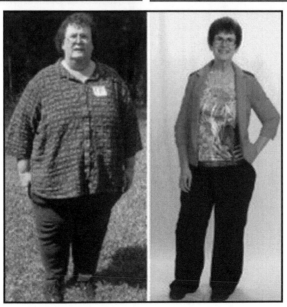

What's next?

I am so grateful for what God has done for me. Living free from food addiction has changed my life. I want to share what I have learned and give you practical steps so you too can be free! The study guide includes:

- Bible study
- Thought-provoking questions
- Creative activities
- More photos
- Action Plan

Please visit
WWW.TERESASHIELDSPARKER.COM/GUIDE
Download the Sweet Grace Study Guide as my free gift to you!

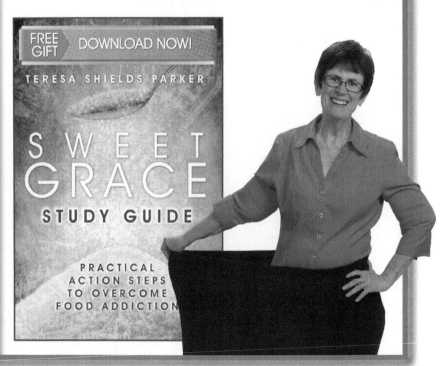